# NEW NURSE'S SURVIVAL GUIDE

# NEW NURSE'S SURVIVAL GUIDE

**Genevieve E. Chandler, RN, PhD**
University of Massachusetts Amherst
Amherst, Massachusetts

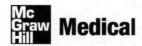

New York  Chicago  San Francisco  Lisbon  London  Madrid  Mexico City
Milan  New Delhi  San Juan  Seoul  Singapore  Sydney  Toronto

New Nurse's Survival Guide

1  2  3  4  5  6  7  8  9  0   DOC/DOC   14  13  12  11  10  9

ISBN 978-0-07-159286-4
MHID 0-07-159286-5

This book was set in Plantin by Glyph International.
The editors were Joseph Morita and Karen Davis.
The production supervisor was Phil Galea.
Production management was provided by Somya Rustagi, Glyph International.
The book designer was Eve Siegel.
The cover designer was Aimee Davis.
The index was prepared by Robert Swanson.
RR Donnelley was printer and binder.

This book is printed on acid-free paper.

**Library of Congress Cataloging-in-Publication Data**

Chandler, Genevieve Elizabeth.
    New nurse's survival guide / Genevieve E. Chandler.
       p. ; cm.
    Includes index.
    ISBN-13: 978-0-07-159286-4 (pbk. : alk. paper)
    ISBN-10: 0-07-159286-5 (pbk. : alk. paper)  1. Nursing.   2. Nursing—
Practice.  I. Title.
    [DNLM: 1. Nursing.   2. Nurse's Role. WY 16 C4553n 2010]
    RT41.C34 2010
    610.73—dc22                                        2009036580

McGraw-Hill books are available at special quantity discounts to use as premiums and sales promotions, or for use in corporate training programs. To contact a representative please e-mail us at bulksales@mcgraw-hill.com.

This book is dedicated to my support team,
Conor, Maura, Michael, and Mark

# Contents

# Preface

*New Nurse's Survival Guide* offers you a lifeline to make the leap from school to practice. You will learn about the reality of day-to-day practice from the engaging new nurse narratives that take you behind the scenes to see what the work of a nurse is really like. The information shared in this book will help you be well prepared for securing that new job and provides you with guidance for managing the professional responsibilities of the new nurse. But first: Where's the job?

Nursing is supposed to be recession proof, right? Also, there is still a nursing shortage, so where have all the positions gone? Nursing may well be recession proof and there is still a nursing shortage; however, many other jobs are being hit by the economic recession. This means spouses are losing their jobs or their hours are being cut back, so nurses are increasing their hours or returning to work. Many nurses are delaying retirement, so there are fewer positions to fill. Like all corporations, hospital budgets are being cut back too. A tighter budget may mean ancillary positions are being frozen, which translates into more responsibility for the nurse but no new positions being opened. You may have to look further than you anticipated or in a different area of nursing. The landscape has changed. This book is designed to assist you in being the best prepared you can be for the job search, the interview, orientation, and not only surviving but thriving in your first year!

This book has the information you need to secure your first position. There is more competition than ever for fewer positions, so you need to know what *hospitals are looking for* and what *you need to bring to the table*. You need to think about how to stand out from all the other new nurse graduates. You need an edge. Your edge is to know what hospitals want before you apply for a job. That is what this book is about: knowing what you need to be successful as a new nurse and knowing what health care facilities are looking for in their new employees. I can tell you up front that all positions, from acute care to home care, are looking for experience, initiative, evidence-based practice, and leadership.

1. What can you do to gain on-the-job experience while you are in school?
2. How can you demonstrate that you are a nurse who takes the initiative to be involved?

3. How do you base your student practice on evidence?

4. How have you demonstrated leadership?

## Experience

Look into any type of position that will give you a leg up in health-care experience. Can you work as a CNA? Are there student nurse positions available? What about summers? Vacations? You may have made more money in your past summer job, but health-care experience will open doors for your future career.

## Initiative

Hospitals are interested in nurses being involved in shared governance, serving on committees, and volunteering for councils. Taking initiative in patient care is key. How have you been an advocate while you were a student? Do you have a track record of being involved in your school? Are you in the Student Nurse Association (SNA)? Have you been an SNA officer? Are you on school committees? Are you an honor's student? Have you collaborated on faculty research? Have you received scholarships or awards? These activities have put new grads out ahead in the job search. In recent experience, those students who took the initiative to be involved in school were the first to land positions in facilities of their choice.

## Evidence-Based Practice

All facilities: acute care, rehab units, and long-term care need to base their nursing practice on evidence. Researching the evidence should be second nature to you. Let the interviewer know what you can do, how you have used evidence as a student, and how you have shared evidence with practicing nurses.

## Leadership

All nurses are leaders, or at least that is what your new job will expect. How have you demonstrated leadership as a student? Did you take the lead to work with faculty on research projects? Did you challenge the way things were done and use the proper channels for change? Health care knows it needs to make massive changes to be affordable and accessible. How can you demonstrate that you know how to negotiate and lead a change?

The narratives in this book with help you plan your job search and anticipate how you will survive and thrive in your first year of practice. Now, more than ever, you need to know the inside story so you can move into your new career well informed and positioned for success!

Chapter 1 is designed to help you reflect on your original ideas about being a nurse and help you begin to consider how your dream and the reality of nursing work and life fit together.

In Chapter 2 there are questions for you to consider in reflecting back on your experience with life's transitions so you are well prepared with the information and energy needed for this major leap from school to practice.

Chapter 3 is all about how to construct your cover letter and resume so you will be invited on interviews and then know how to prepare for them.

Chapters 4 and 5 review the basics of what you need to remember from your training as a nurse so you can demonstrate your facility with the two essentials of patient care: triage and safety.

Chapters 6, 7, and 8 have insights and critical information that have never been shared before from nurses in their first year of practice: the bonding necessary to make it, the culture that you need to look for to survive, and the journey that surviving the first year will entail during your first year out of school.

Chapter 9 lets you know how far you will have come after a year in practice, and finally, Chapter 10 presents viable options for what's next.

# Acknowledgments

I'd like to thank my friends and colleagues Beth, Lisa, and Caroline for their wonderful contributions on the central importance of patient safety, the essentials of triage, and the necessity of a winning resume and interview.

- Elizabeth A. Henneman, RN, PhD, CCNS, FAAN, is an Associate Professor School of Nursing at University of Massachusetts, Amherst, Massachusetts. She is a brilliant and treasured colleague, who insists in this serious role we have that is central to patient health and safety, there must be some fun or none of us will last!
- Lisa Wolf is a clinical assistant professor at the University of Massachusetts, Amherst School of Nursing, and a practicing emergency nurse. She teaches both pre-licensure and registered nurses what to do first in a variety of settings. Her area of research is triage and clinical decision making.
- Caroline Gould is assistant director for career planning at the University of Massachusetts at Amherst and serves as the career advisor to the School of Nursing. She has also been a psychotherapist, a public school teacher-trainer, an art archivist, and a shellfish warden, among other things.

I am indebted to the investment and commitment of the First-Year Study research team for their congenial collaboration, creative contributions, and collegial connections that produced the personal narratives that are at the heart of this story.

- Lisa Buckley, RN, BS Second Bachelors graduate
- Nancy Craig Williams, MS, RN, PhD candidate
- Jan King, MSN/MPH, DNP expected 2010
- Regina Kowal, DNP expected
- Jan Thouy, RN, BS, RN to BS graduate

# How to Use This Book

This book is your mentor, your guide, and your own coach for moving from school to practice. This book is designed to be interactive, with pertinent questions for you to answer to assist you in increasing your self-awareness so you can demonstrate your ability on job interviews and in your new position.

**To get the most out of this book:**

1. Answer the questions as if we were having a conversation.
2. Read the stories to learn what is expected of you and what you can expect from you new boss and new peers.
3. Take the information seriously. Review triage, assessment, competencies, and leadership. Your interview is your opportunity for the job to get to know you. When you go with the right information and are prepared with good questions, you will feel more confident and present yourself as knowledgeable, self-aware, and passionately invested in nursing.
4. Read and remember the three essentials, bonding, culture, and journey, to survive and thrive in your new job.

Get out your highlighter and be prepared for eye-opening recommendations so you can get the job you want and be the nurse that you have worked so hard to be.

# NEW NURSE'S
# SURVIVAL GUIDE

# CHAPTER 1

# The Dream

By attending and graduating from a nursing program, you have been prepared as a nurse to be in a place of honor, to witness and care for individuals and their families who are struggling with illness and striving toward health. You are the nurse who is on the front line with individuals who are extremely vulnerable, along with their worried families and frightened friends. You are the RN. Welcome to nursing!

You have worked hard for two, four, or five years to become a nurse. You had a dream when you applied to school that you would make a great nurse. And you will! Now it is time to make that dream a reality. Nurses are needed in all areas of practice. You can choose a job that fits your interests, your needs, and your lifestyle. This is a great time to graduate. Although shortages fluctuate, there are plenty of positions open in many areas of the country. In finding the right job, you are in the driver's seat. You can choose where you would like to work. So where do you begin? To learn about your own interests, start by collecting the information on what you already know. Jot down your responses to the following reflections to begin developing a plan for your move into the professional world of work.

 **Reflection 1: Begin by recalling the original dream that pulled you through nursing school.**

- In your dream of being a nurse, where did you see yourself working? In a hospital? In a community setting? In home care? In hospice care?

- Who did you imagine taking care of? Babies? Kids? Adults? Elders?

- When you were in nursing school, in what areas of clinical did you feel "I can do this!" or "I like working here."?

- What type of nurse did you meet and think, "I want to be just like that nurse."? What was that nurse like? What was that nurse doing?

- And the perennial question we all wrestled with: "Should I get med/surg experience or go right into the specialty I love?"

My good friend Susan, the most competent, patient-centered nurse practitioner I know, recently offered sage advice to new grads looking at different options for their first position. Susan wrote,

*I don't think hospital med-surg nursing as a "base" holds up anymore. Every area of medicine is so specialized now that I'm not sure any one serves as a great qualification for any other. Neither are they liabilities. Any work you do will help you mature as a nurse and help you learn how to make decisions. Being a good nurse is about gathering clinical experience and smart decision making. Every clinical experience will build on your previous experience. One of the best nurses I work with now worked in a development office before she became a nurse at age 35. Then she worked on a surgical floor at a major teaching hospital for less than a year and is now with me at school. She could move into any kind of new situation and be a great nurse, even with the so-called limitations of her background. She is smart, fun, funny, and has a great attitude. If someone put her in the ICU with a good mentor, in 6 weeks I would let her take care of my dad. Attitude and brains translate and transfer to any clinical specialty.*

Read Susan's words again. It contains very important guidance for your job search. Now you are getting a feel for reflecting on what fits with who you are. What about where you want to practice?

Start by considering these factors:

1. Geographic area
   a. Small town, big city, rural, urban?
   b. What part of the country?
   c. Can you move? Why not?
2. What facilities are in the geographic location you have chosen?
3. Is there a magnet hospital, that is, does the hospital that you are considering have the American Association of Colleges of Nursing

(AACN) magnet designation, signifying it is a work environment that attracts and retains nurses? (For more details on magnet designation, see Chapter 8.)

4. Can you go directly to a specialty area of your choice?
5. Is there adequate orientation to prepare you for the specialty?
6. Is there a designated residency program where there are planned introductory activities for 6 months to a year? See Chapter 6 for information on residency programs.
7. How long do you have your own preceptor?
8. What happens when your preceptor time comes to an end?
9. How is a nurse evaluated?
10. What is indicative of an excellent evaluation? Certifications? Continuing in school? This is really asking the question "What does this organization value?"
11. How is a nurse promoted? Is there a designated career ladder?
12. How does a nurse move up the career ladder?

These 12 questions are great topics to discuss during an interview. Chapter 3 describes the interview process in more detail.

# BUT FIRST: TAKE A BREAK!

School is hard, intense, and there is a lot of pressure to perform. Nursing students have consistently reported that the rigors of learning what it takes to be a nurse were far beyond anything they could have imagined. Although the end result of all that blood, sweat, and tears is positive, the education process does take a toll on your brain, body, and spirit. Give yourself a rest and reward after it is all over. Figure out what will work for you: getting a job and then taking a break or taking some time for yourself first so you can look for a job when you are more relaxed and have renewed energy. Sarah, after graduating from a 4-year baccalaureate program, strongly recommended taking a break between school and work so you can begin refreshed and ready to go:

*School was a rat race. There was so much pressure among peers during that last semester, and e-mails were flying back and forth: "Where are you applying?" "Have you heard yet?"*

Sarah admitted that the buildup of the job search, filling out applications, hearing about friends going on interviews, and some even getting job offers was absolutely overwhelming:

*The feeling of terror began in the senior seminar, our professional role class, when we met with a nurse recruiter last March. At that time we asked, "When should we apply?" The recruiter responded with, "You haven't applied yet?"*

The pressure builds. When Sarah was getting ready to graduate she recognized that she needed a break, time away from school, a reprieve from the job search, and a diversion from nursing too.

*After I graduated I went with my mom's church to Mexico. I began sending job applications in from there. Sitting on the plane on the way back I thought, "I hope I have not heard anything; maybe I am not ready." School was an emotionally demanding time. After reflecting on how exhausted I was, I decided to take time off. Nursing is so intense. I needed to renew my energy and spirit.*

Taking time for yourself is not easy in any job market if you do not know where you are going next. You have to trust you are going to land on your feet and you will find a job when you are ready. Feeling ready means being relaxed and refreshed. With the attrition rate for first positions up to 60% in the first 6 months, we can safely say many new grads are not ready and accept positions that do not fit.

Sarah suggested a test question to see if you need a break: "Right now, do you feel ready to start nursing school again?" If you gave one of the following responses: "No!" "No way!" "Never!" then you probably ought to consider taking a break because starting a job means starting classes again and beginning a new clinical, without faculty backup.

It is so hard to be in the middle where you have no idea what you are doing. Bridges (1980) recognizes how vulnerable we are during transition, when the past has receded and the future has not yet arrived. This is the same for any job. If you don't know where you are heading next, it is difficult to relax. Nurses, however, are in a good place. Whenever you decide to look for a job, you will find one. However, currently we are getting mixed messages with the fluctuations in the economy and the threatening shortage of nurses, so it may be more difficult to find the ideal position. The first job may not be on the unit you dreamed of, so if that is the case, consider starting in subacute, long-term care, or rehab, where you will get good experience and your first year under your belt. You'll be more successful looking at potential positions and making career decisions if you have some experience beyond school. Check out what Sarah did:

*The family my mom and I stayed with in Mexico said, "Come back anytime." So, when I got back to Boston I decided to return to Lua, outside of Mexico City. I justified this wild decision to myself by saying that I would get to learn Spanish. But once I got back I needed structure, so I volunteered at the high school in the English learning lab. I really like to teach, so I enjoyed it. I created activities around their favorite music (which is our popular hip-hop), and it was very rewarding.*

With time and distance away from the job search crush, Sarah also was able to get some perspective on what she wanted to do next. Like everyone else in her class, she had considered Boston for a job move but decided to go back to Colorado where she had spent part of her childhood.

*While in Mexico I searched online and found out that the University of Colorado was a magnet hospital. I applied and went to find an apartment.*

You, too, want to make sure you land in the right place. That is the key: the right place, the place that fits for you. To make this important career decision, you need to collect data and compare your findings. To make a decision, create a list to compare attributes of each position you are considering. You have many options.

## Reflection 2: Questions for You and the Job

I. **You'll want to look at positions closely.** Start with location:

Where is the facility located?

Where can you afford to live?

What is the transportation?

Consider the cost of parking, rent, food, and the local gym.

**2. Consider the specialties available.**

Table 1-1 describes numerous specialty options for new graduates.

**3. Don't be shy when inquiring about the position you are applying for.**
You want to cut down on any surprises after you accept the job.

What is the job description?

What are the shifts?

How are preceptors decided?

How is the nurse manager described?

How is the staff described?

When can you tour the unit?

**Table 1-1.** RNs with an Associate's (2-year) Degree or Bachelor's (4-year) Degree

| Practice Area | Description | Web Site |
|---|---|---|
| Medical/surgical nursing | General nursing | American Academy of Medical-Surgical Nurses, www.medsurgnurse.org |
| Labor and delivery | Families and infants | www.awhonn.org |
| Postpartum | Families and infants | www.awhonn.org |
| Neonatal intensive care | Families and infants | www.nann.org www.awhonn.org |
| Pediatrics | Working with newborns to 18-year-olds on a general pediatric unit or a specialty unit such as respiratory, neurology, pediatric intensive care unit (PICU), or pediatric rehabilitation | http://www.pedsnurses.org http://www.pediatricnursing.com www.napnap.org |
| Perioperative | Operating room | www.aorn.org |
| Emergency nurse | ER education, certification, and research | www.ena.org |
| Orthopedic | Education certification and research | www.orthonurse.org |
| Oncology | Cancer nursing | www.ons.org |
| Critical care | Intensive care nursing | www.aacn.org |
| Gerontology | Caring for the older adult | www.ngna.org |
| Rehabilitation | Caring for patients in rehabilitation settings | www.rehabnurse.org |

*(Continued)*

**Table 1-1.** RNs with an Associate's (2-year) Degree or Bachelor's (4-year) Degree (*Continued*)

| Practice Area | Description | Web Site |
|---|---|---|
| Long-term care | Caring for patients in long-term care facilities and nursing homes | www.ngna.org |
| Hospice | Palliative care nursing | www.hpna.org |
| Home care | Visiting nurses | www.vnaa.org |
| Mental health | Psychiatric nursing | www.apna.org |

**4. Get the details of orientation.**

How long is the orientation?

What is involved? Are there straight classes (new grads report that too many classes may be too much information, too fast), or are classes and clinical integrated?

Will you have a preceptor?

What is the support system after orientation (typically orientations last from 6 to 12 weeks; some places assign mentors after orientation, and some have a year-long new grad group).

Use the worksheet in Figure 1-1 to compare possible job opportunities.

| | Hospital 1 | Hospital 2 | Hospital 3 |
|---|---|---|---|
| Geographic area? | | | |
| Cost of living? | | | |
| Position Shift? | | | |
| Salary? | | | |
| Manager: Open, friendly, interested? | | | |
| Staff:  Welcoming? | | | |
| Teaching? | | | |
| Supportive? | | | |
| Orientation:  How long? | | | |
| What is involved? | | | |
| What happens after orientation? | | | |
| Is there a new grad program? | | | |

*Figure 1-1.* Evaluating prospective jobs.

You are a precious commodity. Yes, you. But for your first position, you may not get your preferred shift. In fact, most new nurses start on nights. Many find that after the initial shock wears off, the quieter atmosphere on nights offers an opportunity to work at a slower pace and in a less chaotic environment than days. Mary reported that nights gave her time to think through her care, consult with her preceptor, and look things up. Plus, in her facility a clinical resource nurse was available who was extremely helpful. On nights Mary had time to learn from the resource nurse.

Days, 12-hour shifts, nights, weekends, and holidays are all new experiences for the beginner. Research describes that managing family expectations and job requirements can sometimes be conflicting and stressful for the new nurse (Fink, Krugman, Casey, & Goode, 2008). Working holidays is a new experience, but I always found holidays a very special time to be with patients.

Mary describes her holiday shift:

*Thanksgiving night, a time for food, wine, family and festive merriment—and I was going to work. Times like these it is really crummy to be a nurse. Not only was I working on the holiday, but was also working the 12-hour overnight shift. Welcome to the bottom of the seniority ladder! My large cup of milky coffee in hand, and with plenty of healthy nibbles to get me through the small hours of the night, I resigned myself to a long, but probably enjoyable, night on the mother/baby side of our Birthing Center.*

*Day shift could barely manage to blurt out a cursory report before they flew out the door, off to their family and friends; better late than never. With the report I had that night, I may very well have had a unit full of golden retrievers for all the information I received from the day shift, but I could understand their excitement to go home and enjoy the holiday. First things first. I wanted to eyeball these ladies, their new babies, and put faces with the names and see if anything seemed amiss. Walking down the linoleum-tiled hallway, my practical nurse shoes squeaking delicately, I reflected that the patients probably wanted to be stuck in here even less than I did, so I had best try to make the evening tolerable, if not the most entertaining of Thanksgivings. Eight newly delivered mothers, some with one baby, one with two, and the lady all the way down the long dim hallway with her little one in the neonatal intensive care unit (NICU) up on the seventh floor.*

*Room 628 was as far away from the nurses' station as a room could be on this particular unit, and it was the last room I stopped in on my introductory rounds that night. A polite rap on the door, and I stepped in smiling cheerfully to introduce myself. Something wasn't right in that room. Something about this woman reminded me of my old med/surg patients, not the fairly healthy women I work with every day.*

*Concern and anxiety tried to wrap their clammy fingers around my neck, but I shoved them away to be dealt with later. Dawn was this woman's name, and everything about her sent warning signs tingling through my body. She looked wrong, sounded wrong, and Dawn knew something wasn't right even if she couldn't identify the source of her discomfiture. Not a young mother,*

*Dawn was 36 years old according to my scrawled notes, but her pale, sweaty, swollen face, and raspy, gurgling respirations made her seem ancient. Anxiety was traced through every line of her being, but not for herself.*

*The first question I had from Dawn was "How is my baby?" All I could think to myself was that I didn't really care at that precise moment because we had more immediate things to worry about. With a calming breath I suggested we call the NICU and speak with the nurses there about her tiny 4-pound son. Stepping closer to dial the phone for her I could hear the wet, coarse sound of her breathing, and those cold fingers of worry squeezed at my heart; had she had any trouble breathing today, I asked her. "All day," was the answer as she took the phone from my hands. Dawn was nodding and her face was less tense as she held the phone to her ear and spoke with the nurse upstairs.*

*I took my centering breaths and focused on how I was going to get this woman well, or at the very least, the help she needed. As she talked on the phone I wrapped the blood pressure cuff around her arm and collected the all-important vital signs: respirations, pulse, blood pressure, and when she was off the phone, her body temperature. Dawn's respirations were rapid and shallow, like she just couldn't catch her breath, her pulse was rapid, and her blood pressure was high, too high, frighteningly high. The NICU told Dawn that she was free to come up and see her beautiful boy as soon as I gave her the OK. Every fiber of her being wanted to leap from that bed, race to the seventh floor, and hold her child, but she could not go, might not even survive the trip, might never see her son again if we didn't get the fluid from her lungs and her blood pressure under control. So I told Dawn that we must wait, that her pressure was too high and that her lung sounds were too moist, and that her physician must come see her before she could go upstairs. Soggy tears rolled down her pretty, puffy face, and I tried to comfort her—partially for her emotional health and partly because I was afraid she would have a stroke if her blood pressure went up any further.*

*I raised the head of the bed, placed a pillow under her right shoulder, and dimmed the lights. "No TV, no boisterous visitors, and please don't try to get up" were the instructions I left her with as I placed the call bell in her swollen hands.*

*I flew down the hall to call her obstetrician, and as luck would have it, I spotted him in the hallway waiting for the elevator. Relief flooded my body, and*

*I called out to him to wait. Irritation flickered across his face, and he placed his foot in the elevator to hold it as he turned to me. I provided a clear and succinct report of Dawn's symptoms, how she was so frighteningly similar to my old congestive heart failure patients, and so very out of place on such a basic postpartum unit. I was graced with a parting sneer, and the order to give her 100 mg of metoprolol to help lower her blood pressure, and with that the elevator door slid shut in my dumbfounded face. He wouldn't listen to me, but I knew I had to help Dawn.*

*I gave Dawn her blood pressure medication as the doctor had ordered, and I called up to the NICU to take a few Polaroids of her baby. Thirty minutes seemed like an eternity, but eventually they passed. I took her blood pressure again, and it was even higher than the first time. I immediately put a page out to Dawn's doctor, but I also took matters into my own hands.*

*I notified the charge nurse of the situation, and I initiated a "rapid response" code that would bring a critical care nurse and a respiratory therapist to my patient's bedside for a thorough assessment. Within minutes they were there, and when the doctor called me back 40 minutes later, I was sure to mention their presence and their great concern over Dawn's condition. He would be there in 10 minutes, and then there was a dial tone. Do they teach rudeness in medical school?*

*I went back to Dawn, and I brought her the snapshots of her son. I spoke soothingly to her while they drew blood for lab work, and I helped her splint her abdominal incision with a folded blanket when she coughed her wet, wracking cough. We talked about her other children, and we called her husband and asked him to come be with her. I wiped the sweat-plastered hair from her forehead, and I emptied the urine from her Foley catheter bag. We sat together and waited for the verdict.*

*When her doctor arrived there was a brief conference between the obstetrician and the hospitalist, and before I could finish checking on my other patients, they were whisking Dawn away to the intensive care unit (ICU). In the end Dawn spent over 2 weeks in the ICU, received more than 7 units of blood, and required intensive follow-up care with a cardiologist. I went several times to visit Dawn on the ICU, and I was sure to bring her new photos of her son, or one of his blankets for her to hold, each time I saw her. I don't know if it meant anything to her, but I always think of that Thanksgiving night when I have doubts about why I am a nurse.*

Holidays? Weekends? Nights? Sickness does not have a clock. It arrives on its own time. Fortunately, you will be there to assess patients and advocate for their needs. You will be there to make sure the patient has the proper care, just as Mary did.

You are the connection between health and illness, you conduct the assessment, recognize the symptoms, and anticipate the intervention. You are the connection between life and death. So the place you work needs to have nurses who work as a team, consult with one another, help each other out, and are open to your questions and concerns. Consider all your options.

# CONCLUSION

You have worked hard to get to where you are, and the next step is to land in the right place. "Land" is an appropriate term because with the rush at the end of the semester, the celebrations of graduation, and the pressure to find a job, it feels like you have been catapulted into a new life. To land on your feet, take a breath, and read on. You are more in control than you think.

## References

Agency for health care research and quality (AHRQ) (2007). Nurse staffing and quality of patient care. Retrieved July 1, 2009 from http://www.ahrq.gov/clinic/tp/nursesttp.htm.

Bridges, W. (1980). *Transitions*. MA; Addison-Wesley Publishing Co.

Fink, R., Krugman, M., Casey, K., & Goode, C. (2008). The graduate nurse experience. *Journal of Nursing Administration, 38*(7-8), 341–348.

# CHAPTER 2

# The Reality

Get ready! To be prepared to start your first job as a nurse, you need to have the energy and enthusiasm that it requires to make this amazing life transition from student to nurse. One way to prepare is to take some time to reflect on your style of making a life change. Take time to sit quietly, just think about how you have managed transitions in your life so your old ways can support your new career rather than get in the way. To assist you with understanding how this move from school to work will affect you, this chapter offers essential information about the process of transition but most importantly, it gives you the opportunity to apply the theory to yourself. Transition is one of those things like swimming. I could spend pages describing how to properly swim the backstroke but if you never get in the water you will never learn the backstroke. To best prepare yourself for your future you need to apply these insights about the transition process by answering the questions about how you make a change. Come on in, the water feels fine!

## TAKING THE LEAP FROM STUDENT TO NURSE

We like to think of going from a student to a nurse as a transition. The word *transition* implies an orderly, predictable process that one can easily follow. Good idea, but according to new nurses, not the reality! A recent graduate wrote that "learning how to be a nurse is more like a giant leap into the unknown than a transition." The actual details of the nurse's role are related to the specific position you accept and the people you work with. How one responds to the move from student to nurse is determined by each unique individual. We are not machines that automatically go from one developmental step to another. We each are very different in our approaches to change. Yes, of course there are general stages that we go through with every role change. For example, the *honeymoon:* "Yay! I am out of school, can finally be a nurse, and actually get a paycheck!" The *shock/rejection:* "Whoa! I know nothing, don't know anybody, don't even know where to park my car!" *Assimilation:* "OK, I can do this. Just get organized, put one foot in front of the other." To finally, *acceptance:* "Yes! I have my own patients, I can assess, I can ask questions, I can spread my wings. Oops! Where'd my preceptor go?"

You have done this before. Think about it. You went off to college by yourself, found a new job on your own, and made new friends. You just have to reflect on how these four role transition stages apply to you to recognize and even predict and prepare for how you will respond to this huge transition.

## Reflection 1: Going Off to College

Although you have experienced other life transitions in the last few years, the one we have in common is going off to college, or for some, going back to college for a second degree. That was a major change, to leave home or leave a familiar career. Everyone went through the high of the honeymoon phase, "Yeah! I made it, I got into nursing school!" to the low of the shock phase, "Oh no, I am in, but look at all this work!" Yet in each stage, we each handle the experience differently. Evidence from research on life transitions tells us that as a group we go though similar stages differently, yet as an individual we each go through our own life transitions in a similar manner (Bridges, 1980). So if you think back on your transition to school, you will be able to anticipate your reaction to beginning your first nursing position. These questions focus on going off to college for the first time, an experience that 2-year grads, 4-year grads, and second-degree students all have in common.

Reflect on your unique reactions to going off to school, what it was like for you to go from high school (or from a community college or another major) to college.

1. How did you react to your first month in college?

2. How did you family react to your first month in college?

3. Reflect on the feelings you had about starting a college program. Jot a few down.

4. Who was that first friend you made? How did that happen?

5. How did you learn to manage all the work?

6. How did you manage to still have a life?

_____

The reactions you identified to beginning a new life in school, how you responded to your family, and remembering the feelings you had (overjoyed to leave town, then sad you left) will help you anticipate your reactions as you move from student to nurse. Once you arrived at school, developing a new support system of friends, finding mentors in older students and faculty, managing all the schoolwork, and establishing a social life were probably similar to how you will manage this new transition from school to work, *unless* you consciously plan on doing something different.

Developing a conscious transition plan starts with reviewing how you have managed other transitions in your life and identifying what you'd like to alter about your approach to change. The research tells us the way we each manage life's transitions started in our childhood (Bridges, 1986).

*I hate to think that the way I handle changes as an adult is based on how I managed change as a child because I didn't. I was a wreck going off to kindergarten. I didn't handle change well at all; change managed me. My mother and my teacher, Mrs. Delaney, can both attest to my little 4-year-old head down on my desk sobbing during morning cookies and milk. Of course, as an adult, I handle change differently. I am more mature. Maybe. Come to think about it, the experience of entering graduate school was not so different! During my first week back to school, listening to the first lecture on nursing theory, I thought I was in a foreign language class. I did not know what the professor was talking about standing down in the pit lecturing seventy students. Then when she assigned all that reading for homework, I panicked! I didn't exactly cry, but I felt like putting my head down on the desk and sobbing. I instantly went from the honeymoon stage to shock/rejection. At the morning break I called my former boss from the lobby of the school of nursing to beg for my job back. Fortunately, she wisely suggested I give graduate school more than one day. So, judging from my experience, maybe there is something to this theory of each of us having our own unique way of handling (or not) transitions. It's worth thinking about.*

Going from student to nurse is a *big* change. Not only does this move from school to work involve your transition into the professional world, but you are also jumping off on your own from a sheltered college life to supporting yourself both financially and socially. I know that if you are a senior you have been counting down the days, but take a moment to consider how you have made transitions in your life so this stage will be less frightening and more predictable.

What is transition all about? You have studied human growth and development. You know about the stage of moving from adolescence to adulthood, leaving school, going off on your own, supporting yourself, right? You know that no matter at what age you go through a school program and move into a new job, the school-to-work experience is a leap of faith. Believing what you memorized, practiced, wrote about, and were tested on will somehow provide you with a base to take care of the complex, multisystem illnesses in several patients is a leap of faith. However, even though we intellectually know this should all work out, we still need to engage in the experience on a practical and emotional level. We still need to find a new place to live, go to an unfamiliar place to work, work with people we don't know, make new friends, *and* deal with the emotions that are brought up by leaving a familiar place, an established routine, and people we are comfortable with. Now it is your turn to reflect on your own experience. What is really going on here? This whole transition from student to work will be more manageable if you take a moment and reflect on how you personally handle transitions. You have been through them before, you know your style, so let's make your approach to transition transparent so you know what to expect next.

## *Reflection 2: Leaving the Routine*

1. When I think about leaving my friends in my nursing program, I feel . . .

2. When I think about leaving the school routine (after you yell, "I CAN'T WAIT!"), what will you miss about being on campus, being in class, and being in between classes?

3. When I think about not having faculty to rely on, I feel . . .

No matter how joyful you are about never being assigned 200 pages to read in one night or how relieved you are not to have to write a 20-page care plan, leaving the familiarity of the school routine and your peers is both a joy and a loss.

*When I graduated from my undergraduate program I could not wait to get out of school. I mean, we counted the days from some time in February on a roll of paper towels that hung from the ceiling of the cafeteria from 100 days to graduation. Then, something strange happened. When the end finally arrived, we stayed. After families left graduation weekend, we stuck around to pack up, or at least that is what we told our parents. But before any suitcase was opened, my six best friends and I climbed up the steel green fire escape ladder to the flat pebbly roof above the fourth floor of Mary Margaret Hall. We had never done this before because Buffalo snow does not melt until mid-May and as undergraduates we took off right after the last final. But graduation was a week later, so we actually experienced our first western New York spring. With blankets, water bottles, and baby oil in tow, we settled into beach mode up on the roof. Under the clear blue sky, we spread out our blankets and camped out. After the 100-day party celebration, the stay-up-all-night to make floats for the MUD (Moving Up Day) parade, and semiformal at the Sheraton, the graduation practice, the annual pub crawl, the family brunch, and finally the baccalaureate ceremony, we still couldn't leave each other. Those were four hard years of study, party, exams, party, clinicals, party, best friends, boyfriends, and now, before we even left the campus, a huge wave of nostalgia rolled over us. Lying there in a row, Sarah, Katrine, Marybeth, Winnie, Gio, and I stared into our futures and reminisced about the past.*

I did not know at the time this postgraduation nostalgia was called *termination*. But the termination process of reviewing the past, reflecting on good times and bad, and anticipating the future but proceeding with caution is a healthy part of the leave-taking process. As I stated earlier, we are vulnerable in times of transition when the past is receding rapidly and the future has not yet arrived (Bridges, 1980). That is exactly what it feels like: The past is going and the future is not here, so you are caught in between. What can you do? When you are feeling vulnerable, you need to take care of yourself and keep good friends around. Now it's your turn to reflect.

1. How do you usually take care of yourself? List a few familiar routines:

2. As Deepak Chopra (1989) reminds us, we need to stay in balance. When things are stressing you out, what do you do to keep a balance?

3. Who do you talk to when times are tough?

It is important to recognize that the transition experience is normal. To move successfully into a new role, typically you pass through the four stages of role transition: honeymoon, shock/rejection, assimilation, and acceptance. I think our 100-day ritual back in college was the honeymoon. We had all the symptoms of the honeymoon stage: high energy, eternal optimism, confidence, invulnerability, and incredible relief. Looking back, I think our trip to the Buffalo beach up on the roof was a ritual of preparing us for honeymoon to shock! Now what? Transition takes time and energy. It requires courage. Now it's your turn to reflect.

Recall a time when you were celebrating an important ending.

1. What was the ending?

2. Where was it?

3. When was it?

4. Who was there?

5. What was it like?

6. What was the reminiscing about?

7. Recall a good ending where there was recognition and celebration.

8. What do you have planned for your own graduation?

# FROM ENDING TO BEGINNING

You have probably already had some coaching on searching for a job, creating a resume, and going on a job interview. Chapter 3 addresses these important issues, plus the career services office at your school can be an enormous help. Right now, though, what is important is learning what to look for that will make this transition work for you.

We put together a top research team of an RN-BS student, a second bachelor's student, a PhD, and a DNP student to go out and talk to a sample of novice nurses in their first year to see what was going on out there. The aim of the study was to develop a thorough description of the novice nurses' experience of the first year of practice to assist graduating seniors and new grads, educators, and practicing nurses in mentoring new nurses through the transition into practice. When *the First Year Study research team* analyzed the data by putting the new nurse stories together and looking for patterns, the results identified three important themes: *bonding, culture, and journey.*

1. Bonding: You cannot become a new nurse on your own; you need to feel *bonded* to your new team. We can tell you what to look for and how to choose a place to work.
2. Culture: You are coming into a whole new *culture* that is nothing like you have experienced before. We can let you know what to expect.
3. Journey: You must recognize that this process of entering will not happen in the first week, first month, or even in the first year. Becoming a professional is a *journey* and we can tell you what to look for.

Schlosser and Waldo (2006) studied the new nurse transition and recognized that the new grad needs to know that transition to practice is difficult and "should not be misunderstood as a failure on their part or a sign that you are in the wrong organization or even in the wrong profession" (p. 49). Understanding the transition process is essential so you can feel more comfortable during the difficult times by recognizing you are not the first one to experience this process, you are not in this alone, and the more you know about the process the better you will fare. That's a promise.

# WHAT YOU NEED TO KNOW

The new graduate will enter a resource-poor environment with staffing shortages and an increase in patient acuity, demanding sophisticated assessment skills, initiating clinical interventions, using management skills, and demonstrating leadership capabilities. The attrition rate of new nurse employees has been reported from 20% to 60% during the first year of practice with only 9% of registered nurses younger than 30 years old and 25% of nurses retiring in the next 5 years (Griener & Kneble, 2003). This means you need to find the right place to work the first time around because a wrong job fit is both stressful for you and costly for the employer. All new hires need to find a fit so they can grow and learn while feeling safe and appreciated. To take on your first job as a nurse, you will need to feel passionate about your workplace and the people you work with. Nothing less will be able to successfully support this transition from student to nurse. Finding a facility with values similar to yours, accepting a position on the unit that feels like a match, and making sure you have adequate orientation and supervision is key.

# WHAT YOU ARE EXPECTED TO BRING WITH YOU

Something very exciting is happening between practice and education, and you are the center of attention! Hospitals and schools are collaborating on describing the Nurse of the Future by defining the competencies required to practice nursing. This is a first. It is groundbreaking to have practice and education work closely together. This pioneering effort began in 2003 when the Institute of Medicine (IOM) (Greiner & Kneble, 2003) identified five areas that all health-care professionals need to focus on to be prepared for today's work environment:

1. Delivering patient-centered care
2. Working as part of interdisciplinary teams
3. Practicing evidence-based medicine
4. Focusing on quality improvement
5. Using information technology

Being a recent graduate, you most likely know about these areas of focus. Nursing leaders have stepped up to define how each category is applied in nursing. The Quality and Safety Education for Nurses (QSEN) project built on the knowledge and skills identified in the IOM report with the intention of educating nurses to continuously improve the quality and safety of the health-care system (Cronenwett, Sherwood, Barnsteiner, Disch, Johnson, Mitchell, et al., 2007). In several states schools and hospitals are partnering to develop a description of competencies necessary to become a new nurse. The competencies are divided into the knowledge, skills, and attitudes necessary for the new nurse to be successful. For example, QSEN defines patient-centered care as "recognizing the patient or designee as the source of control and full partner in providing compassionate and coordinated care based on respect for patient's preferences, values, and needs." One of the knowledge components of patient-centered care is to be able to "describe how diverse cultural, ethnic, and social backgrounds function as sources of patient, family, and community values," with the skills necessary to "provide patient-centered care with sensitivity and respect for the diversity of human experience," and the attitude to "recognize personally held attitudes about working with patients from different ethnic, cultural, and social backgrounds." This sounds a lot like school, doesn't it? Don't turn off yet! *It is vital for you to know what hospitals are talking about before you walk into an interview.* You are the nurse of the future, so you want to know what hospitals, home-care agencies, and long-term care facilities are looking for in interviews. Visit the QSEN web site at http://www.qsen.org/competency_definitions.php, see what they expect, and learn the language being used so you can be part of the conversation.

At this point, education, both 2- and 4-year programs, are examining their curriculum to make sure the competencies are covered. Hospitals are developing transition programs based on the competencies to support the new nurse's entry into practice. The QSEN project is designed to serve as a resource to guide curricular development for academic programs, be a map for hospital programs that are designed to assist the nurse in transitioning to practice, and provide ideas for continuing education programs. As you are moving into the job market, it is critical to know what nursing practice is focusing on for the new grad. Review the QSEN site to become familiar with the information and language used to describe the competencies of the nurse of the future. Some hospital leaders are talking about individualizing new grad orientation to fit with the knowledge, skills, and attitudes the new nurse brings into practice. You can prepare for orientation by considering the knowledge, skills, and attitudes you learned in school and what you still need to learn on the job so you are able to demonstrate that you are aware of your own learning needs. Look into whether your state has developed its own nurse of the future competencies. Several states have very informative Web sites. Oregon has created an education-practice collaborative to better prepare nurses to meet the needs of an aging ethni-cally diverse population (check out http://www.ocne.org/). Vermont has developed an initiative to coach new nurse preceptors with a Web site packed with excellent resources for new nurses, including information on improving communication, managing conflicts, and developing competen-cies at http://www.vnip.org/links.html. A must read! With jobs being more competitive, you can be prepared for your interview by demonstrating an awareness of the competencies you feel comfortable with and those you need to learn. Hospitals don't expect you to know everything but they do expect you to be aware of your own learning needs.

# TRANSITION

## Where Will You Work?

By the time you have made it to senior year, you have some ideas about what nurses do, where they work, and what might interest you. A wonder-ful aspect of being a nurse is that when you graduate with a generalist degree from a basic program in a community college, you can choose to work in a variety of units in the hospital. Or with a baccalaureate degree, you also have the option of working at a magnet facility, in a public health agency, or in a position in the military, like Brie.

*After graduating with a BS degree I felt confident and well prepared to go out and do what I had always dreamed of. I was excited to begin my career. At that time I could never have imagined I would do or see the things I have in my first 3 years in nursing.*

*First, I received my commission in the U.S. Navy and went to Officer Indoctrination School for 5 weeks. After completion I was stationed at the National Naval Medical Center in Bethesda, Maryland, the flagship of navy medicine. I was placed on the surgical/trauma ward, and this is where I began my nursing career, taking care of causalities from Operation Iraqi Freedom and Operation Enduring Freedom.*

*I truly feel blessed and privileged to have been given the opportunity to work with and care for our nation's true heroes. Each and every one of these young men and women has touched me in different ways.*

*I remember like it was yesterday the first time I truly connected with one of our injured soldiers. I had him as a patient the night he was transferred from the ICU to the ward. He was still in rough shape. This patient was an Army Special Forces officer with 16 years of service, injured in Iraq by an IED blast. He was blinded, had multiple fractures that left him immobile, several soft tissue injuries, and shrapnel peppering his whole body.*

*It was a very difficult night for him. He was dealing with intense pain and having flashbacks that brought him back to the very moment when he was injured, to when he lost two of his men, and to where his life was changed forever. Because he was blind, which left him to live in darkness, and he was unable to move his extremities, he could not wake himself from these flashbacks/ nightmares. I remember sitting at his bedside holding his hand, praying with him, and crying together. We got through that night, and I continued to be his nurse for the few months he remained with us. He and his wife and I have become close friends, and I have been with them during some of their very low times of recovery. I have also been able to witness some very high moments. I was there when he finished the Marine Corps marathon and Army 10-miler, being one of the first to run these races blind. He has truly inspired me and showed me the meaning of perseverance.*

*Working with these men and women everyday, being at their side when facing challenges and seeing them make great strides, has been quite the experience. I have realized this is why I joined the military. There is no way to describe the feeling I get when I see an amputee patient walk back on to our floor with his new legs to say hi, or when a traumatic brain injured patient comes back from rehab talking, or when a patient who had a gunshot to the face can start eating again. Nursing has been so rewarding.*

New graduates have many options. You will start as staff nurse and move up the clinical ladder. Many organizations have clinical ladder programs where you must meet certain criteria to be promoted from Clinical Nurse 1 to Clinical Nurse 2. Nursing used to be thought of as having a flat, horizontal career trajectory where you could only move sideways to another clinical position if you wanted to stay at the bedside. If you wanted to move up in title and salary, you could choose an education or management track. Now there are more options to creating a career path within the clinical setting (see Table 2-1).

There are many different positions in each faculty to learn about, so you know what resources are available.

**Table 2-1.** Nursing Positions in Acute Care Facilities

| Position Title | Position Description |
| --- | --- |
| Staff nurse | Works at the bedside with patients and families, a central part of the health-care team, usually assigned to a certain shift but may rotate between shifts. |
| Resource nurse | An expert nurse in a certain clinical area or may rotate throughout the facility. Some organizations require resource nurses to have an advanced degree in their specialty (e.g., medical nursing, mental health nursing, cardiac care, etc.) so they are called clinical nurse specialists (CNS). Some organizations have a resource nurse on all shifts, in each specialty. A resource nurse or CNS is an excellent source of support for new nurses. |
| Charge nurse | An experienced staff nurse in charge of a specific shift, i.e., charge nurse for days or nights. |
| Nurse manager | Usually manages one or two units and is the administrator of the unit, the link between your unit and upper administration. Research reports units function best when the nurse manager is approachable, accessible, visible, and influential (Tucker & Edmondson, 2002). |
| Clinical nurse leader | Can be a title assigned to the individual in charge of a shift, or may be the charge nurse, who organizes and supervises the shift. Sometimes the charge nurse position rotates; at other times it is a permanent position with an increase in pay. The clinical graduate nurse is also a specific graduate degree (CNL) that prepares the nurse to function as a case manager or the care coordinator for a particular group of patients, providing direct patient care, see http://www.aacn.nche.edu/Media/FactSheets/CNLFactSheet.htm. |
| Nurse practitioner | An NP requires an advanced degree and clinical experience to be certified as an advanced practice nurse. NPs diagnose and treat a wide range of health problems, emphasizing health promotion, disease prevention, and education; they have their own caseload of patients and function in a variety of settings. The position can require a masters (NP) or doctoral degree (DNP). See http://www.aacn.nche.edu/DNP/index.htm |

*(Continued)*

**Table 2-1.** Nursing Positions in Acute Care Facilities (*Continued*)

| Position Title | Position Description |
| --- | --- |
| Nursing supervisor | A nurse expert who oversees day-to-day operations in the whole facility or a designated clinical area. Usually a supervisor is assigned to each shift. |
| Nursing director | An expert nurse who directs a specific clinical area, such as the surgical director or pediatric director. |
| Vice president | Oversees nursing services and frequently other clinical departments. Same level as other hospital vice presidents. |
| Quality assurance person | Oversees the hospital's activities that are designed to achieve the desired level of care. |
| Staff educator | Directs the in-house education department that designs and delivers education on new programs and reviews programs, policies, equipment, and innovations. |
| Clinical ladders | A promotion, recognition, and rewards system based on clinical criteria that vary in each facility. A clinical ladder program is designed to describe progressive levels of staff nurse responsibilities and expectations from clinical nurse 1 to clinical nurse 5 that is commensurate with salary increases. Facilities design their own clinical ladder to encourage the development of the professional nurse and to meet the needs of the organization. |

# INTEREST IN EDUCATION?

As a nurse you can choose to enter into teaching through the staff education department in a hospital or, if you have your baccalaureate degree, you may consider a graduate program so you can teach in a community college or function in a baccalaureate clinical instructor position. In a graduate program you would specialize in an area such as psychiatric clinical specialist, pediatric nurse practitioner, or nurse midwife. A clinical nurse leader program will build on your assessment, diagnostic, and case management skills to provide you with advanced case management skills. A doctorate in nursing practice, DNP, is the specialty degree that will be required by 2015 to practice as a nurse practitioner. There is the opportunity of being a professor in a university and a nurse scientist by pursuing a PhD. Currently, a growing number of fast-track programs are available to take you from a bachelor of science (BS) to a doctorate (PhD) or BS to DNP. Moving into an administrative career track is another option. (See Chapter 10 for What's Next?)

## Can You See Yourself as a Manager?

Several management positions are available in nursing, as listed in Table 2-1. Many facilities require a graduate degree to apply for a nurse manager position. Consider this possibility once you feel you have a solid clinical base.

# CONCLUSION

Knowing where you are going, how you will mange the journey, and what to expect when you get there can give you a bit more control when everything seems out of your control. Knowing what the organization expects of what you bring to the organization, can empower you to advocate for yourself, and enable you to anticipate the future. Transitions, positions, and possibilities are key to consider. This is a thrilling yet stressful time. Knowing how to manage transitions and having a map of the territory will support you in navigating this exciting world of practice.

## References

American Association of Colleges of Nursing. (2005). CNL fact sheet. Retrieved from http://www.aacn.nche.edu/Media/FactSheets/CNLFactSheet.htm

Bridges, W. (1980). *Transitions*. MA: Addison-Wesley Publishing Co.

Chopra, D. (1989). *Quantum healing*. New York: Bantam Books.

Cronenwett, L., Sherwood, G., Barnsteiner J., Disch, J., Johnson, J., Mitchell, P., et al. (2007). Quality and safety education for nurses. *Nursing Outlook, 55*(3),122-131.

Greiner, A., & Kneble, E. (2003). Health professional education: A bridge to quality. Institute of Medicine. Retrieved from http://www.iom.edu/CMS/8089.aspx

Oregon Consortium for Nursing Education. (2009). Retrieved from http://www.ocne.org/

Tucker, A., Edmundson, A. (2002). Managing routine exceptions: a model of nurse problem solving behavior. *Advances in Health Care Management, 3*, 87-113.

Schlosser, M., & Waldo, M. (2006). The first 18 months of practice. *Journal for Nurses in Staff Development, 22*(2), 47-52.

Vermont Nurses in Partnership. (2009). Links & Learning. Retrieved from http://www.vnip.org/links.html

# [CHAPTER 3]

# Getting a Nursing Job

CAROLINE GOULD

You are going to get a job—there is no doubt about that. There is a nursing shortage, which means there are more job openings than nurses available to fill them. This is partly brought about by the comparatively low pay that nursing instructors earn, leading to fewer professors in nursing schools, followed by fewer students in nursing schools, leading to fewer nurses, thereby putting you in the position of getting a job relatively easily.

But read that first statement carefully: You *are* going to get a job. That's *a* job, not necessarily *the* job you want. Oh, you'll get a job, but it might not be in the city you want, the hospital of your choice, the shift you prefer, your ideal specialty, or the pay rate you feel you deserve. There is competition in the world of nursing, and you may need more than blind luck to find your way to a nursing job that feels as though it fits you well. This chapter offers suggestions on managing your job transitions and developing your career with a little more conscious understanding of the processes going on behind the scenes.

I am the assistant director for career development at the University of Massachusetts, Amherst, and I help nursing students as they take their first steps out into the world with a new diploma and license in hand. I have held many different jobs myself, including a year-long stint on the medical wards of a hospital working alongside nurses as an emotional counselor with the Social Work Department. Through my many job transitions and career moves, I have learned a lot about how to make good work choices and how to present relevant skills and experiences to potential employers.

The more you are able to articulate to an employer the kind of nursing job and environment you will thrive in, the more likely you will be to end up with that job. Knowing what you want will give you an internal guide to help you evaluate potential job situations. The following exercise will help you to be clear about what you want and do not want in your next nursing job.

This is an exercise in gathering information about your perfect nursing job and environment, adapted from Barbara Sher's book *I Could Do Anything If I Only Knew What It Was* (Sher, 1994), that I regularly use in nursing classes.

1. Start by considering *your nursing job from hell*. Take a couple of minutes to write just one or two paragraphs about the qualities of the worst nursing job you can imagine. Flesh out the awful details of one whole day, including when you wake up, how long your commute is, how the shift change happens, the number of patients, the situations you encounter during this awful day at this awful job, and what you feel like when you leave at the end of the day. Be sure to include all the particulars, such as angry patients, demanding bosses, and disgusting smells. You get the idea. (Stop here and do the first step of the exercise. It works better to read no further until you have finished this part of the exercise.)

2. Now it is time to move on to *your nursing job from heaven*. Take your awful job from hell, and detail by detail, flip everything around until you get a positive. Do you hate a long stop-and-go commute? Your wonderful job is a 5-minute, clean, inexpensive public transportation ride away. Hate oncology? Your wonderful job is perhaps a comfortably busy daytime emergency department shift. Twist each bad detail in to a good attribute, and you are on your way to expanding your ability to describe, to yourself and others, what you want in a nursing job.

Whenever I facilitate this exercise with a nursing class, I find a surprising diversity of interests and desires. Some people like a commute as a transition time, lots of nurses don't like maternity or pediatrics, some like being very busy, and others do not. Most people want a respectful environment where they are treated fairly, but beyond that, well, you will just have to take the time to do the exercise yourself to identify more clearly those things you really need and those you really don't want in a working environment.

Your ability to articulate what you want in a job, as well as the skills, experiences, and credentials you bring to an employer will greatly affect your ability to get the nursing job you want. Whether through writing, as in a cover letter and resume, or in person during a job interview, the more you can clearly describe your needs and your strengths, the more in control of the job transition process you will be.

# COMMUNICATING CLEARLY THROUGH YOUR RESUME AND COVER LETTER

Put yourself in your employer-to-be's shoes. They are worried about finding quality, experienced people to solve specific problems at the worksite. They are concerned that their staffing levels stay high, their employees deliver quality service, and any feedback they get about anyone's performance is positive. They are too busy, too harassed, and too necessarily self-involved to take the time to read your resume and cover letter carefully the first time through. They don't care about you—yet. So they won't take the time to read through a rambling cover letter, they won't squint their way through a 9-point, autobiographical two-page resume, and they won't forgive any mistakes in grammar or misspellings. What they are looking for is a clear record of your most relevant skills, credentials, and experiences that quickly informs them how you can solve their particular problem.

## Resumes

A resume is not an autobiography. Let me say it again because so few people realize this. *A resume is not an autobiography.* A resume is a one- (or at most two-) page shorthand description of the education, skills, licensures, credentials, and experiences that are directly relevant to the position you are seeking or to the audience you are addressing. Relevant, relevant, relevant, relevant, relevant—not to you, or your mother, or your best friend, but to the intended audience, such as your next employer-to-be.

Resumes need to state these relevancies both clearly and consistently. People do not read resumes so much as they quickly scan them for the qualifications important to them. And the first look through is often a matter of mere seconds, during which the reader might decide to put the resume in the "looks-promising-read-in-depth-later" pile or the "no" pile. That resume has to catch a reader's eye in a positive fashion immediately. Here are some suggestions to consider as you write or update your resume, followed by some examples (Fig. 3-1):

## *Format*

- Create a Word document resume from scratch. Do not use a "resume template." Most resume readers know the templates, and you will look lazy and uncaring if you use one. Bad way to start.
- Do use boring fonts like Times New Roman and Garamond. They are the fonts used in book publishing, which means our eyes are used to reading them quickly for content. Boring font, exciting content equals good.
- Stick to font sizes between 10 and 14 point, and consider steering clear of italics and underlines (they reproduce and scan poorly).
- Start explanations with descriptive, active verbs, and leave out both pronouns (I, me, they, them, etc.) and articles (a, an, the) for consistency's sake. If you end each phrase with a period, do so consistently. If you don't, then don't—consistently.
- All entries under a heading are expected to be in reverse chronological order, which means the most recent first, followed by older, then oldest. New heading? Start the reverse chronological order all over again.
- Don't waste words on the obvious, but do describe your relevant accomplishments, using numbers where possible.
- Do have a simple professional-sounding voicemail message, and do Google yourself. Any Web entry should be "grandma approvable"— nothing racy or edgy (at least while you are looking for a job).

## *Content*

- The audience for your resume wants to know certain things about you, so hand them those things on the silver platter that is your resume. Your name, contact info, licensure, nursing degree, rotations, other credentials, nursing internships and externships, health-care-related jobs, and community service—all your relevant information has to be easily seen during the first quick read.
- Learn all you can about your audience. Devour any job ad and use the language and priorities of the qualifications/requirements section to reword and rearrange your resume. No job ad? Then look at the mission statement (often under an "About Us" section of a Web site) for language and the main concerns of the employer. If you can't find anything, then do your best and guess what they care about and what they most likely need to know about you. ICU is very different from a

Visiting Nurses Association (VNA) job, and each site will care about different aspects of your experience.

And finally, this all takes a bit of time. Considering that the possible outcome could be a job that could literally change your life around, these few pages are worth all the effort you can put into them. Get lots of feedback, but understand that everyone has a different idea of what a resume should look like and include. In the end, it is your judgment call, your life, and your resume. See Fig. 3-1 for sample resumes.

## Cover Letters

A cover letter is a formal, business-formatted letter that, first and foremost, acts as a routing device for your resume (Fig. 3-2). The first line or paragraph in the letter states very clearly that you are applying for a specific job opening. This helps your resume get to the right desk at the right time for the right job. It is a boring, unoriginal, and effective way to start your letter.

As I have said, people so rarely have time. If they don't quickly see why they have your resume in their e-mail or on their desk, they probably will not take the time to read through the entire cover letter to figure it out. Quick and to the point is the rule of the day.

And yet these application readers are real people, too. This is still a letter to a human being, no matter how formal and distant the connection and process might feel. Although they will spare you little attention at first, it is your job to communicate clearly, concisely, effectively, and yet still be friendly. Not so different from being a good nurse, yes?

Once you have told them what these materials in front of them are about, your next job is to let them know, in narrative form, how you meet their needs. Notice that I do not say you get to talk about how this job would be so good for you and your career. Just the opposite. This second important use of the cover letter is to tell them how your skills, experiences, interests, and passions will help solve their specific staffing problems. Meanwhile you are showing that you can communicate through the written word, just as during the interview you will be showing your skills in good oral communication.

## SUBMITTING APPLICATIONS

Submitting applications all boils down to *doing exactly what they say*. If Hospital A in a major metropolitan city wants you to fill out an online

**Sally Street**
833 Pine Street, Amherst, MA  01002    413-898-4444    sstreet@yahoo.com

**EDUCATION**
**University of Massachusetts Amherst, School of Nursing**
 Bachelor of Science in Nursing, May 2009
 Commonwealth Honors Program, GPA: 3.4

**Springfield Technical Community College**
 Associate in Nursing, May 2004

**CLINICAL ROTATIONS**

| | |
|---|---|
| Baystate Medical Center,<br> Springfield MA | Advanced senior practicum in<br> Medicine/HIV+ |
| Holyoke Hospital,<br>Holyoke MA | Senior HIV/AIDS case study, pediatric<br> component |
| Marks Meadow Elementary<br> School, Amherst MA | Community health<br>Pediatrics |
| Western Massachusetts<br> Hospital, Westfield MA | Medical/Surgical floor; Cardiac floor<br>Medical floor; Psychiatric/Mental Health |
| Mary Lane Hospital, Ware MA | |
| University of Massachusetts<br> Medical Center, Worcester MA | |

**ASSOCIATION MEMBERSHIPS**
National Student Nurses' Association
University of Massachusetts Amherst Student Nurses' Association

**EXPERIENCE**
**Farren Care Center,** Turners Falls, MA        2007–present
 Nurse's Aide  - Provided rehabilitative nursing care to promote and restore independence on both spinal cord and head trauma units. Experience with ventilator-dependent
 individuals, straight catheterization, bowel programs, tube feedings, dressing changes,
 tracheotomy and colostomy care.

**The Atrium at Cardinal Drive,** Agawam, MA     2004–2006
 Nurse's Aide - Provided complete evening care on skilled nursing unit.

**Jerry Lewis Muscular Dystrophy Camp,** Butler, PA   Summer 2003
 Camp Counselor - Assisted campers with ADLs and encouraged
 participation in planned events.

**LEADERSHIP EXPERIENCE**
**Alpha Chi Omega Sorority,** Amherst, MA     2006–present
 Community Service Chair - Organized and participated in activities
 ranging from tutoring children at several local community centers to
 playing bingo with residents of nursing home.
**Habitat for Humanity,** Alternate Spring Break    2008–present
 Fund-raising Chair.
**Sophomore Representative to Clinical Faculty**   2007–2008
 Served as liaison between students and clinical faculty.

**LANGUAGES**
Fluent French, intermediate Hebrew, basic Spanish

**TRAVEL**
Israel, Egypt, Turkey, France, Netherlands, Denmark, Germany, Czech Republic, Hungary, Italy.

*Figure 3-1.* Resume.

**Jim Jones**
900 North Pleasant Street, Amherst MA 01002    jjon@gmail.com    (413) 546-1000

## EDUCATION

**University of Massachusetts Amherst,** School of Nursing Expected: May 2009
 Second Bachelor of Science in Nursing                                Current GPA: 3.72
**University of Pennsylvania,** School of Education, Philadelphia, PA
 Master in Education, School Counseling PreK–12                              May 2004
**Franklin Pierce College,** Rindge NH
 Bachelor of Arts in History                                                May 2000

### Clinical Experiences

| | |
|---|---|
| Center for Extended Care in Amherst MA | Nursing Home 2009 |
| Wing Memorial Hospital, Palmer MA | Medical Surgical Floor 2009 |
| Baystate Medical Center, Springfield MA | Pediatric, Adult Psychiatric, Acute Renal 2008 |
| Holyoke Hospital, Holyoke MA | Maternity Floor 2008 |
| Amherst Bangs Center, Amherst MA | Community Health 2008 |

## WORK EXPERIENCES

**Nursing Intern,** Joint Center, Cooley Dickinson Hospital, Northampton MA    2009–present
• Assess patient health conditions; offer necessary interventions if change in status.
• Include patient and family members in care planning according to patient's health needs.

**Home Health Aide,** Hospice of the Fisher Home, Amherst MA    2008–present
• Implement care for 6 patients with personal care, comfort measures, and meal preps.
• Facilitate patients and family members' spiritual needs and end-of-life care.
• Provided post-mortem care.

**Assistant Residence Director,** University of Pennsylvania, Philadelphia, PA    2004–2007
• Provided orientation to undergraduate staff on university's judicial system, crisis management protocol, and alcohol and drug education.
• Offered crisis counseling and made referrals to academic/mental health services.
• Supervised and trained 18 undergraduate Resident Assistants.

**Personal Care Attendant,** Philadelphia, PA                              2003–2004
• Cared for hypoglycemic child, monitored blood glucose, diet, and feeding through GI tube.
• Provided personal care and comfort to elderly women at home.

## OTHER EXPERIENCES

Volunteered as outpatient assistant; cleaning and dressing wounds for students at the Tibetan Children's Village School's Health Center in India                              2001
Taught English and Social sciences for Grades 7–10 at the Tibetan Children's Village School in northern part of India,                              2000–2003

## AWARDS

U.S. State Department Fulbright Scholarship. 2001

## LANGUAGES

Fluent Tibetan and Hindi

*Figure 3-1. (Continued).*

Barbara Brown
321 Main Street
Amherst, MA 01002
413-546-2345
bbrown@gmail.com


February 10, 2010


Manager of the New Nurse Program
Dartmouth Hitchcock Medical Center
One Medical Center Drive
Lebanon, NH 03756


Dear Manager,


It is with great enthusiasm that I write this letter to apply for the New Nurse Program at Dartmouth Hitchcock Medical Center.


Currently I am completing the internship portion of the Second Bachelor of Science Degree Program in Nursing at the University of Massachusetts at Amherst. I am presently at a small, diverse, and rural Critical Access hospital. We cater to a seasonal influx of skiers, summer campers, second home owners, and all-year residents. I have a concentrated focus in Medical Telemetry Nursing, and am excited about this placement because I know I will be able to use the experience gained here in any area of nursing. I am aiming my future nursing career toward working in the emergency department, but as a new graduate nurse I am quite willing to work in any part of the hospital setting.


My strength is my ability to work both independently and as a team player. For the past year I have also volunteered at a home health agency. The internship has been a rewarding and challenging experience, and it has helped me to develop my skills working with patients recovering at home from surgical procedures.


I believe that with my skills, my enthusiasm for my new profession, and my willingness to learn that I will be a positive addition to your department.


Enclosed is my resume for your review.


Sincerely,


Barbara Brown

*Figure 3-2.* Cover Letter.

**Ruth Rouse**
4 New Plains Road, Erving, MA 01344   413-732-8877   rrouse@yahoo.com


Franklin Medical Center
Human Resources Department
543 Main Street
Greenfield, MA 01301


March 17, 2010


Dear Nurse Manager,


I am writing to apply for a Medical/Surgical or Labor and Delivery nursing position at Franklin Medical Center. I am currently completing a nursing internship on Spoke 4 as a part of my final semester in the University of Massachusetts Amherst's Bachelor of Science in Nursing program. Prior to my internship, I spent a semester on Spoke 3 completing a medical/surgical rotation with Lori Aldren as my instructor.

As a result of the last nine months spent completing clinical hours at Franklin, I am already familiar with hospital policies, CIS documentation, and charting. I have begun to build relationships with doctors, nurses, and assistive personnel. This familiarity will ease my transition as a new employee and will make me a more efficient and effective new graduate nurse.

In addition to my education, internship, and clinical rotations, my nursing practice is informed by my prior work experience as a youth program coordinator in Springfield, MA. I worked with young people from diverse cultural backgrounds facilitating workshops on healthy relationships, sexual health, and substance abuse prevention. These experiences showed me the value of supporting people establishing their own health goals and helping them achieve them. I am sensitive to people's emotions, respectful of their boundaries, and value helping to empower individuals to take an active role in their own health care.

I look forward to discussing the potential for employment at your facility. My resume is included for your review, and I will call you next week to check on the process of this application.


Sincerely,

Ruth Rouse

*Figure 3-2.* Cover (*Continued*).

application where you have to type in each job you have ever held, followed by a block where "You may paste your resume here," well, that's what you do. In fact, please go back into that block, copy your now reformatted resume, paste it back into Word, and make sure it is still readable. If they ask you to give the details of each of your rotations, including the numbers of hours, give them exactly that, in exactly the format they ask for. It may be tedious and time consuming, but very often it is only after you have fully completed an application that they will consider you seriously.

Now Hospital B, off in some rural area, might be happy with a paper copy you snail mail to them—or not. Call the Human Resource Department and ask. In another scenario, perhaps you are at a family gathering and your Aunt Ida loudly demands you e-mail her your resume because she is friends with the CEO at her local hospital. Do exactly that. Plus send a general cover letter stating the kind of nursing you are interested in, along with your resume, as Word attachments (watch out for compatibility issues), and to be safe, perhaps include all that info in the body of the e-mail, as well as sending her a hard copy by snail mail.

As a side note, whenever you send your resume as an attachment, please do not just title the document "Resume.doc." Do you know how many "Resume.doc" files resume readers have in their computers? Put your name in the title, as in "SallySmithResume.doc" or SallySmithCoverLetter.doc." See Fig. 3-2 for sample cover letter.

So the big picture is that you give the employers-to-be exactly what they are asking for, in exactly the format they require, every time. If you are unsure, call and ask. It may be annoying that different sites require different applications, but it is unlikely that every employer will have the same process anytime soon. In fact, the technology both applicants and employers use is constantly changing. *If you are unsure how to send in your application materials, just call and ask.* You want to let them know you can follow directions, so you can move to the next step: The interview.

# INTERVIEWING

Although an interview should never be considered some sort of benign interrogation, neither is it a casual affair to which you can wear your scrubs. Do some prep work before you even head out to the interview, and it will help you to project confidence as you head toward your first professional nursing job.

Learn what you can about the environment and the job you are interviewing for. Look up the hospital and the unit on the web. Google any names of people you know you will be meeting with. You don't want to look like you have not done your homework  about the situation you are interviewing for—that's just plain rude.

Then you need to refamiliarize yourself with your resume. What, exactly, are the experiences in your life that are most relevant to this job? Your nursing internship or rotations, sure, but what about some community service where you helped out at the local senior center or the time you assisted at a Relay for Life? These kinds of experiences can speak to familiarity with particular populations, such as working with elders or breast cancer survivors.

Come up with some questions for the employer. Write down five or so to bring along because if you don't have any, you run the risk of appearing dumb or uninterested. Here are some examples:

- What are the qualifications of individuals who have excelled in this position?
- What is your nurse-to-patient ratio?
- During the orientation phase, will I have just one preceptor or many? How long is the orientation?
- How long has this position been vacant?
- What are the call requirements for this position?
- What type of person are you seeking?
- What will be the measurements of my success in this position?
- Are there professional developments or continuing educational opportunities?
- What are the next steps in this application process?

*But don't ask about money until they are offering you the job!* They are probably going to pay you the going rate for the position and the geography, so concentrate on getting the offer, and then worry about the money.

Finally, prepare for the day. What will you wear? Hopefully it will be some version of clean, moderately formal, conservative clothes, with no overpowering odors of any kind. Later, after you get the job, you can be the snappy or sexy dresser you feel you are. But for now, you want the interviewer to focus on your answers and experiences, not your earrings or your bellybutton.

Bring along a folder or portfolio with an extra copy of your resume, a list of your references, and perhaps even an unofficial copy of your transcript.

They may not request them, but there will be points in your favor if they do ask and you have them. Oh, and leave your cell phone behind. There is that sickening moment when an interviewee reaches for that phone—and then turns it off. Phew! Don't even let the employer's stomach start lurching. Leave it behind!

Be early. Not on time, and never late. It is way too difficult to recover with even reasonable excuses for tardiness. Just make your mind up now to be 15 minutes early. Be nice to everyone, even the lowliest aide, orderly, and receptionist. Always stand when you shake hands, even if the other person doesn't. And it is OK to take time to think about your answers and to ask for clarification if you didn't understand anything they said.

They will probably ask you questions about your experiences with teamwork (the good and bad parts), your work ethic and attitude, your ability to connect with patients while maintaining professional boundaries, and your communication skills. They will be listening for specific examples from your experiences because most recruiters base their questions on the idea that past experience very often predicts future behavior. But be careful of a couple of areas:

- Don't bad-mouth anyone, ever! Even if you have had the most evil boss, professor, or manager in the hemisphere, this is the wrong time to go on about it. It is very unprofessional behavior to disparage anyone in front of someone you don't know. The interviewer is just going to be left feeling that as soon you are out the door you are going to badmouth her, too.

- This is not therapy. Don't drone on about any marriage, child-care, or other personal issue.

- And once again, leave pay and benefits discussions for after they have offered the job to you, which might be after a second interview. At that point they have an investment in you, and because of that you now have some bargaining coin you didn't have earlier in the process.

Research on interviewing points out some amazing trends in hiring. It all boils down to: *people hire who they know, and people hire who they like.* The world does not seem to follow the maxim of "The best person for the job gets the job" but rather, "Hey! I like you! Want a job?" This then implies that if you want a job, and you don't already know the interviewer, it is a darn good idea to help that interviewer quickly come to like you during your time together. Bring a respectful but friendly attitude, which includes being confident, comfortable in your own skin, present, and accessible. Have you ever noticed how people who are scared are incredibly self-involved? Manage any fear you have so you can be obviously interested in the job, the interviewer, and the environment you are in.

## Thank-You Letters

Yes, you *should* do them, and no, most people *don't* do them—and therefore you can use this to your advantage. There is no lack of stories of people up against stiff competition who got the job just because they sent thank yous. Look at it this way: professionalism. A thank-you letter is a professional communication, and by sending it in no more than 24 to 48 hours after the interview, you are demonstrating a professional attitude and the ability to continue that attitude at a time most people become lazy.

These letters are not long, and they can be in all sorts of format, including e-mail. I know that most student nurses would rather send e-mail because it is what they are used to, and it is easy for them. E-mail is better than nothing. But that nurse manager you met was probably at least a generation older than you, and e-mail is often seen as a throw-away communication. Whereas when I look around my office I still have thank-you cards I probably should have thrown out ages ago but haven't. Here's the rule of thumb: The more effort it takes you, the more effect it has on the audience.

## The Stomachache

There is sometimes no way to avoid the bad timing that comes when struggling with offers-in-hand versus offers-soon-to-come. Say you interviewed with Hospital M first, and while you are waiting to hear from them, you interview for your dream job at Clinic C. Hospital M contacts you and offers a good salary, a signing bonus, and relocation money, but Clinic C hasn't even returned your calls for updates. This is a stomachache, and there is no magic pill or technique to make it turn out all right. Respectfully ask for more time from Hospital M, try to get through to Clinic C, and always stay cool, calm, and professional. At least on the phone. Let Clinic C know there is another hospital interested in offering you a position but you wanted to interview with them before you made your decision. With this line you have already started negotiating.

## Negotiation

Everyone wants to know the magic formula for negotiating the highest salary and the best benefits. Here it is: *a high degree of comfort with risk.* That's it. There is no doubt that by bargaining for more salary or benefits than the employer initially offers, the risk is they say no and move on to candidate number two. That is why you should wait to discuss money and benefits until after you have shown them, in the interviews and every communication thereafter, your friendly, respectful, relevant professionalism. In short, you want them to fall in love with you, so that they *must* have you, no matter the cost.

Do your homework by looking at typical salaries for the kind of nursing job you are searching for. Google "nursing salaries," or go to salary.com to find what a typical salary in the geographic area where you are looking should be. You will need to project complete confidence that you are worth what you ask for, and it is that "complete confidence" factor that usually ruins it for most folks. If you decide to push the envelope, no cringing allowed. Fall apart afterward. While you are preparing, don't forget to consider benefits, professional development opportunities, relocation assistance, a 6-month salary review, and the growth potential of this particular job.

Finally, there is always an emotional amount of money you will need to consider in any situation. Say your dream job at Clinic C comes through. You will be working with the population and health issue you are most excited about, with a clear growth track, on a day shift with an easy commute in a city you can't wait to explore. *But* they offer less money than Hospital M, who will reward you handsomely for taking a night shift in a bad part of town. What is involved here is both the stomachache and your negotiating courage. Just make sure that whichever you pick, you don't start hating the job your second week there. There is not enough money in the world to make up for the bad job where you have to spend some 40 hours a week.

# NURSING CAREER FAIRS

Find career fairs by checking in at your school's Department of Nursing and/or search for "nursing job fair" on the Web. Each fair could be slightly different, so pay attention to any rules about registration. Sometimes the event producers give lots of ideas about how an applicant should prepare, but if not, some basic suggestions follow.

Research the companies that will be there ahead of time. Sometimes the list of who is coming will be posted days in advance, and other times you just have to wait until you are onsite and read the program. Come up with a prioritized list, and most importantly, plan on visiting your number three or five first, to get the jitters out of the way on a less crucial target.

Follow the interviewing guide described earlier for dress, behavior, and attitude. Bring that folder with an appropriate number of paper resumes, and carry it in your left hand because you will be shaking a lot of employer hands with your right.

Come up with a quick two- to three-sentence introduction stating your name, when you are getting (or received) your degree and licensure, and what kind of nursing situation you are looking for. Perhaps you can work in a question about that facility that shows you have done some research. If you are really stumped, find a booth that has a line waiting to talk to the recruiter, and eavesdrop on a recruiter/applicant conversation ahead of you.

Don't be put off if they tell you that you need to apply online, even if they take your paper resume. If the organization receives federal funding, they may have to prove that every applicant was treated exactly the same. It has nothing personal to do with you.

Consider sending a follow-up thank you to the recruiter after the fair, that is, if they give you their contact info.

# YOUR OWN CAREER DEVELOPMENT

Oops! You ended up in the *wrong* job. You thought you loved working with children, but find you hate pediatrics where most of the time you are working with stressed-out, anxious, and angry parents rather than cute and cuddly kids. Oops! You took the higher paying job only to realize more money was the only way that hospital ever got anyone to work in such an awful environment. You have basically two choices.

## Grow

Look at either changing the environment in some fashion, changing your-self, or maneuvering your way into another situation with the same employer. Take advantage of all the continuing education or professional development opportunities available, transfer laterally, and/or apply for other jobs within the same hospital. Remember, people hire who they know and who they like, and looking for a transfer, a promotion, or a different job within the same setting that already knows you is usually easier than starting cold somewhere else.

## Go

No nurse recruiter or employer expects you to remain with them forever. But if I was reading your nurse resume and saw a change of job every 6 months for the past 2 years, well, why would I assume you would stay with me any longer than that? It costs companies a lot of money to hire nurses and get them acclimated to a new situation. If you have a track record of taking off after a couple months, then I probably won't care how skilled or earnest you seem, I'll probably pick someone else perhaps less experienced who might stay a year or five. But if you change jobs at longer intervals, I'll know that you are responsible yet interested in growing and learning.

# YOU ARE YOUR MOST INVESTED CAREER PLANNER

You can request advice from your preceptor, a mentor, Mom, or another family member. You will, of course, talk with your peers and colleagues. You can seek out a professional career coach. But in the end, your future is up to you. Be careful about thinking that putting your nose to the grindstone and just waiting for that recognition or promotion to happen all on its own is going to work. Everyone is busy: you, your nurse manager, and the CEO of the hospital. If you want more, different, or over there, pick your head up every now and again to figure out your path. Watch how other people advance, who gets the promotions, and where your most interesting work is going on. Network with peers and potential mentors through professional organizations and at professional conferences. Be your own advocate.

# CONCLUSION

You really can do this. The skills involved in job transitions—resumes, cover letters, interviewing—are not rocket science. Once you understand what employers are looking for, once you have tailored a resume or two, you'll see that all this stuff is easier than the easiest college class you ever took. Paying attention to what the audience needs can also feel empowering during an otherwise anxious situation. Hopefully this chapter will help you cope not only right now, but with any other job transition in your future. I wish you the best of luck as you reach for your heavenly nursing job.

## Reference

Sher, C. (1994). *I could do anything if I only knew what it was.* New York: Doubleday.

# CHAPTER 4

# Triage and Priority Setting

LISA WOLFF

*"I have six patients to report on," says the off-going nurse. "Mr. Jones is post-op and withdrawing from alcohol, Mr. Smith's BP is dropping and there are no CCU beds, Mr. Brown's wife is standing in the hallway demanding to know when he's going home so she can schedule the cleaners, Ms. Green is a patient with asthma who was extubated yesterday, and I just got a transfer from the telemetry unit, but I haven't gotten to see her yet, although the report from the unit said she's fine."*

Holy cow! What's the priority? Who do you need to see first? How can you keep your patients safe when there's no instructor around? You can use the principles of assessment and triage to order your care, keep your patients safe, and not lose your mind.

## WHAT IS TRIAGE?

Triage is a way to describe how that nurses decide what gets done first. It's a term derived from the French word *trier*, meaning "to sort, sift, or select" and is usually used in the context of disaster or emergency nursing. Triage is based on *assessment*—yours and that of other nurses.

# WHEN DO YOU PERFORM TRIAGE?

The answer to this question is "all the time." Every minute of every shift you are making decisions about what to do next. For example, you pick up your patients at 7 p.m. After taking report from the off-going nurse, you need to make some important decisions. What patient needs to be assessed first? What task should take precedence: medicating patient A for her 4 in 10 pain or finishing the discharge paperwork for patient B to free up the bed for a waiting patient from the emergency department (ED)?

This is a very conscious process in the beginning, and so it may seem mysterious to you to watch an experienced nurse go about her shift almost without obviously considering her options. This is a great time, while you're on orientation, to ask your preceptor to verbalize her process, or "think out loud." Why are you doing that first? Why are you seeing this patient rather than that patient? Why are you choosing to do paperwork before more patient care? If you start off by letting your preceptor know you are trying to "pick her brains" rather than questioning her judgment, you will probably get more thoughtful, complete answers to your questions.

# WHAT ARE SOME TRIAGE SYSTEMS?

Quite a few triage systems are in use in EDs: The Emergency Severity Index (ESI), the Canadian Triage and Acuity Scale (CTAS), and the Australian Triage Scale (ATS) are a few of the most commonly used. What they share is a five-level system that guides the nurse in deciding who needs to be seen first and who can wait. The scales go from "1," a patient who needs to be seen immediately, be resuscitated, or is in critical condition, to "5," a patient who can wait a long time, has a minor injury or illness, and is classified as nonurgent. Most of the time, patients who are "1's or 5's" are fairly easy to identify. It is the patients in the middle who are the most difficult to sort out. Similarly, you may have a very sick patient, an about-to-be-discharged patient, and three "middle" patients in your section or district.

Another way to set priorities is to use Maslow's hierarchy, which you may remember from your mental health nursing or human development coursework. The hierarchical model, usually drawn as a pyramid, starts with the base: physiologic needs like food, air, and water. These correspond to the ABCs of nursing: airway, breathing, and circulation. You cannot progress to higher needs until these basic needs are met. The pyramid then moves upward to safety, love and belonging, esteem, and self-actualization, needs that are important but ones that come after the patient has an airway, is breathing, and is perfusing well.

## The Take-Home Message

When you are thinking about what the patient needs, or which patient needs to be seen first, focus on the ABCs or physiologic needs before considering anything else. For example, you can't worry about your patient's self-esteem or spiritual distress needs until you've made sure she has a patent airway, effective breathing pattern, and good circulation. Similarly, the patient who needs case management gets in line behind the patient with no BP, no matter who is yelling louder.

# HOW DO YOU SET PRIORITIES USING TRIAGE SYSTEMS?

Compare Maslow versus ESI, for example:

Step 1: Consider acuity: Who among your patients is a potential high-acuity patient (a "2")? That person gets checked first.

Step 2: If all patients are of roughly equal acuity, who's being discharged? To where? Does someone need that bed? He or she gets attended to first.

Step 3: If all patients are of equal acuity, the one whose needs are lower (closest to the base) on Maslow's hierarchy gets seen first.

Use the alphabet (ABCDs) to gauge acuity:

**Airway:** Is your most important assessment and therefore the assessment you do first. If your patient is not breathing, stay with your patient and call for help. If your patient is cold and not breathing, call for help anyway.

*Vital signs are important but more important is looking at the patient. I see nurses all the time "getting the story" from the ambulance service and not really looking at their patient. You have to look at your patient. —Lisa, ED nurse*

**Breathing:** Is your second assessment.

- Is your patient working hard to breathe?
- Is his color normal?
- Does he seem anxious? *A restless patient needs to be evaluated not restrained!*
- Is your patient using any accessory muscles?
- Can he speak in complete sentences?
- What is the breathing rate and rhythm? Is it normal?
- What do his lungs sound like? Are there any adventitious sounds? Where? What do you think is causing them?

**Circulation:** The best measures of cardiac status are level of consciousness (LOC) and urine output. These two measures indicate how well the brain and kidneys, respectively, are being perfused. Because these two organs receive about 25% of blood flow each, constant assessment of these two systems is crucial to stay on top of your patient's perfusion status.

**Cardiac output = stroke volume × heart rate:** To keep cardiac output stable, the body will respond to a drop in blood volume or pressure (stroke volume [SV]) by increasing the heart rate (HR). Therefore, one of the first signs that a patient is hypovolemic is *tachycardia*, not a drop in BP!

Ask yourself the following:

- What does this patient look like overall (LOC, color, anxiety level, urine output)?
- What is his HR?
- What does his pulse feel like (strong, weak, regular, irregular)?
- What is his BP? Is he within his trend?
- Does he have any complaints of dizziness or weakness? Fatigue?
- How does his skin look? Are there areas of mottling? Is it warm? Cold?
- Does this patient have peripheral (pedal and radial) pulses?

If this patient is tachycardic:

- Does he have a fever?
- Is he anxious or restless? If so, what is his arterial oxygen saturation ($Sao_2$)?

- Does he feel short of breath?
- What is his heart rhythm?

**Disability (Neurologic):** LOC is the most important part of the neuro status check. In essence, every time you go into the room and interact with your patient, you are doing a neuro check.

Ask yourself the following:

- Is my patient awake? Alert? Responding to my questions?
- Is my patient able to have a conversation without wandering? Is my patient speaking clearly, using the correct words for things?
- Is my patient moving all extremities? If I ask him to squeeze my hands, is his grip equal bilaterally?
- If I ask him to push down on my hands with his feet, is his strength equal bilaterally?
- If my patient is allowed out of bed, is his gait normal? Is he wobbly? Is he walking into things?
- *Most importantly: Is there a change since the last time I interacted with this patient?*

*I set my priorities by the sickest patient first, then prioritize what care I'll give that patient based on their ABCs, and that's not always easy. For example, I had a patient who had both CHF and sepsis. His BP was really low, and I had to get it up with fluid, but too much fluid would have killed him. I give the liter bolus of normal saline the doctor orders, then I listen to the lungs—crackles rising! Aack! I'm drowning this guy! I thought to myself, OK, now what? The patient had a good airway, an O₂ saturation of 98% on 2 liters of oxygen, but rising crackles, although no respiratory distress. I went to my charge nurse, who pointed out that the patient was maintaining respiratory function but wouldn't last much longer without a BP. I spoke with the doctor, placed a Foley, titrated the fluids to maintain an appropriate MAP, and started some antibiotics and vasopressors. —Liz, ED nurse*

*Whether you do assessment by body systems or "head to toe," the most important, yet most difficult part of being a new grad is developing your own system of assessment. Personally, I do my assessments by body system. I do this based on ABCs being in the emergency room. —Lisa, ED nurse*

# HOW DO YOU GET ENOUGH INFORMATION TO PRIORITIZE ADEQUATELY?

To prioritize your care, you need to have some sense of what's going on with your patients: what they've been like over the last shift, are they trending up or down, what specific issues need to be addressed, and what the plan of care is. For example, this is a report you may get at the end of a busy day:

*Mr. Smith is an 80-year-old man admitted for pneumonia. He has a history of atrial fibrillation and diabetes. He hasn't gotten out of bed today because I was too busy with my other patients, and anyway he's going back to his nursing home tomorrow. I think he still has some oxygen on, and he's fine.*

So what's the problem with that report? You really don't know enough about the patient to decide whether he really is "fine" or not, do you?

## Things to Ask for in a Report

- Name, age, diagnosis, MD (the one you're going to call, not the one who hasn't seen him in a week), activity level, diet.
- Presenting complaint.
- Tests done and tests pending.
- Meds given in ED (if recently arrived) and meds that need to be given before the end of the shift.
- Orders.
- Admitting/discharge paperwork done.
- Vital signs throughout the shift, and important changes (improvements or decompensation) and what's been done about it.

## Things to Clarify If Possible

Those things the nurse tells you "need to get done," like paperwork, a bath, a treatment, or dressing change, does he or she mean before the patient goes home? Before the nurse goes home? Before the patient's family arrives for visiting hours? Try to clarify timelines as best you can.

**Discharges:** When is the patient supposed to go? Where? By ambulance? Who needs to be called?

**New admissions:** Has anyone actually seen the patient? Sometimes, if a patient comes to the floor at change of shift, the offgoing nurse doesn't see the patient, and the oncoming nurse won't get to them for hours, based on the ED report, not what the most recent assessment on the floor has been. *This is very dangerous. Always clarify when a patient has last been assessed!*

**Meds for 8 a.m. or 8 p.m.:** Sometimes the off-going shift is responsible for 8 o'clock medications; sometimes it's the oncoming shift. Ask about them so you know they're there. Otherwise you may find out about them at 10 or 12.

## When You Don't Have Any Information at All

It's always crucial that you see the patient you don't know anything about *first.* Murphy's law dictates that that's the patient who will be much sicker than you thought! This can be the patient who's about to be transferred as well. I remember a night in the intensive care unit (ICU) when the report I got on a patient was that "she's all packaged and ready to go to the floor. Everything's fine—they'll be up to get her in 10 minutes." That of course didn't happen, and after assessing my first patient I thought I'd check in on my "stable, ready-for-transfer" patient. She was pale, with crackles up to her shoulders, Sao$_2$ of 85%—the patient had gone into pulmonary edema—who knew when? She ended up staying awhile longer in the ICU. I never accept a report like that again, unless the transferring nurse plans on staying until the patient goes.

## How to Make Sure Your Information Is Correct

- Assess the patient.
- Verify orders and check for new orders.
- Check the medication administration records for accuracy.

*Don't live in the chart! The answer is in the room!* I have a friend who calls nursing a "contact sport"—you have to interact early and often with the patients, not the charts. Check your *patient first.* Make sure your assessment matches what you've heard in the report. However, patients change fast. Just because the off-going nurse didn't hear crackles in the lungs at 6 a.m. doesn't mean they won't be there at 7:30 a.m.

# How to Decide Whom to See First

Consider these potential problems:

**Airway**

Known dysphagia

Cerebrovascular accident (CVA)

Altered anatomy (trach [tracheotomy], gastrostomy [G] tube, nasogastric tube [NGT])

Altered mental status

Craniofacial trauma

Intubated

**Breathing**

Pneumonia

Asthma

Thoracic trauma

Pulmonary edema/CHF

Broken ribs/surgical site pain

Large abdomen/ascites/hepatomegaly/advanced pregnancy

Head injury; brainstem

Patient-controlled anesthesia (PCA) narcotics

**Circulation**

Recent surgery

Gastrointestinal bleed

Recently postpartum/postmiscarriage

Trauma

Postcatheterization

Increased/decreased BP (trend)

Increased/decreased HR

Decreased urinary output

**Disability**

Diabetic (hypo/hyperglycemia)

Substance abuse

CVA

Hypoxia

Sepsis

# THE IMPORTANCE OF ACCURATE, TIMELY VITAL SIGNS

In my research with rapid response teams, the most striking thing I find when I do a chart review is the huge amount of empty space where vital signs should be. As nurses, we make triage and treatment decisions (what this whole chapter is about) *based on clinical data.* That data in its purest form come from physical assessment, patient subjective information, and *vital signs.* If you're not taking them frequently enough, you may not spot signs of deterioration until it's too late. If you are not taking them accurately, it's the same problem. Accurate vitals signs may require you to match the presentation of the patient against the numbers you're getting.

For example, when I was a night educator, more than once I was called to evaluate a patient who was tachycardic (in the 120s or so) and tachypneic (30s). I'd get to the room and listen to the patient's lungs. In putting my hands on the patient, it was clear that the patient was febrile. Very febrile. I'd ask what the last temperature was, and inevitably be told it was 98.6 °F. How was it taken? Orally. The patient was mouth breathing in the 30s so an oral temperature was not going to be accurate. But the nurse didn't put the hot, flushed skin together with the tachycardia and tachypnea because the temperature was "normal." Rectally, the patient had a temperature of 105 °F. Suddenly, everything started to make sense. The lesson here is to always ask yourself, "Does this make sense? Do these vital signs reflect what the patient looks like?" Especially if someone else has taken those vital signs, like a tech or an aide, this is crucial.

## The Importance of Trends versus Absolute Numbers, or When Is a Systolic BP of 80 Good? When Is a Systolic of 110 Bad?

It's really important to get a sense of your patient's history, and their likely compensatory mechanisms or lack of them. For example, you'd think that a systolic BP of 110 is pretty good, right? After all, everyone should have a BP of 110/70 if they're in good shape.

However, let's look at the following scenario:

*Mr. Jones is a 78-year-old man admitted for a urinary tract infection. He has a history of coronary artery disease and diabetes, as well as hypertension. He takes aspirin, metoprolol, and metformin daily. You see his most recent vitals are as follows: BP 110/60, HR 70, RR 24, Sao$_2$ 95%.*

Do these numbers actually tell you anything? Not really. As emphasized in the preceding section, you need to put together the vital signs with the patient presentation. But you want to keep in mind a few things.

Like 75% of people older than 75 years, your patient has hypertension, so his BP probably runs on the high side, even with medication. For this patient 110 is probably quite low. Another thing is his medication. Metoprolol is a β-blocker, which slows the heart rate. That means that when you consider hypotension, you're also looking for the compensatory mechanism, tachycardia, which will not be evident given the β-blocker. Not so easy now, right?

The crucial piece is to put together what you know about the patient, with their history and medications, and then think about what you expect to see. If you don't see what you're expecting, start looking for why you're not seeing it. Thinking this way will help you pick up on issues early, before the patient starts decompensating.

So when is a systolic BP of 80 good? When you've started at 50 and the patient is getting better. Look at the past 24 hours of vital signs. Look at where the vitals are going, and intervene or support accordingly.

Similarly, the patient who needs your immediate attention is usually the patient who is trending dangerously or in a direction you don't like. If vital signs are changing, think, is this a good direction? Is there a reason for this change (e.g., you've given medication, oxygen, fluids, or changed activity level)? Is your patient in pain?

# PAIN AND WHERE IT FIGURES IN

In most emergency triage systems, a pain scale rating of 7 or above out of 10 puts the patient in a more acute category. The patient with pain that is:

New; wherever it is, but especially if it is head, chest, or belly pain

Refractory to the medication they are receiving

Different from their "usual" pain if they have chronic pain

Triggered by some different activity (for example, if Mr. Jones always complains of hip pain after his physical therapy but today is complaining of pain after you've moved him) should have a quick assessment, and a quick call to the provider for further direction

## How to Organize Your Assessments So You Pay the Most Attention to the Sickest Person

To figure out who I need to see first, I use this formula: Complaint + past medical history = potential problem. For example, the patient with pneumonia or chronic obstructive pulmonary disease (COPD) being actively treated for a respiratory complaint gets seen quickly because the patient is already compromised and probably has less reserve. Thus this patient has the potential to decompensate more rapidly. The patient with a cardiac disorder who is showing evidence of difficulty breathing, weakness, or chest pain gets seen quickly. The patient who is postop and has just been medicated for pain gets seen less quickly, whereas the patient with no pain management for hours gets seen very quickly.

Stick with your priorities. If the complaint plus the history results in a compromise to airway, breathing, or circulation (yup, back to the ABC's again), the patient is a top priority. Decibel level of complaint doesn't make someone more acute (besides, if they are yelling, they've got an airway and they're breathing).

## Meds First, Treatments Second, Baths Third, But Colace Is Not the Most Important Med

It's difficult at first not to get caught up in the "tasks" of nursing, like bed baths, linen changes, and medications. All the things you may have been evaluated on in nursing school are based on your ability to complete a task in a timely, accurate fashion, so that's something you may end up carrying over to independent practice. What's different now is that there isn't necessarily anyone who is going to challenge your judgment on which of those things need to happen first.

The concept here is that nursing isn't actually a series of tasks. Rather it's *a series of assessments* and the clinical response to the data you collect in those assessments. If you organize your care this way, you will begin to see the purpose behind all those "tasks," and you'll remember the assessment behind them even if the actual task cannot be completed.

For example, if your patient is very weak, and tells you that he is too tired for a bath, you need to remember that the *assessment* is to check circulation, range of motion, and skin integrity. Can you do that without giving someone a bath? Of course. But part of the reason we do daily bed baths is to do those assessments. If you'd forgotten that, and (reasonably) didn't want to tire out your patient even more, those assessments might not get done.

Giving medication is similar. You need to know what the patient is being treated for, what the "back story" is, and the medications given for those more chronic conditions so that you can figure out what to give first.

I was working with a student one day, and the student's patient was supposed to get about 15 medications at once. The patient had to take her medications with applesauce and was convinced she could only take three spoonfuls of applesauce at any given time. Considering those constraints, what we needed to do was figure out that, if we could only get six pills into her at a time, which of the medications should we give first? So we looked at the list: an antibiotic, some BP meds, an oral hypoglycemic, lactobacillus, Colace, and multivitamins, among others. What assessments did we need to do before we could decide? We needed a lot of information! Full set of vital signs, BP and heart rate trends, blood glucose, last BM, white count. We pretty much had to go through the chart and assess the patient thoroughly in order to prioritize a med pass. And so do you because the tendency is to give the medications in the order they appear on the medication administration record, not necessarily in order of importance.

## How to Keep Your Priorities Straight

It's really easy to get pulled all over your district by the little things: A family wants to talk to you, you have to call a physician, a medication isn't where it's supposed to be, or a colleague is having trouble. The patient or coworker who wants to keep you at the bedside can also completely derail your organization.

Consider what are the most important assessments and responses you need to do for each patient. For patient A, who has pneumonia, you need to check mental status, lung sounds, and make sure antibiotics and respiratory treatments are given. For patient B, with a diagnosis of urinary tract infection (UTI), you'll want to check mental status, urine output, and BP and make sure antibiotics are given and fluid balance is maintained. Sometimes it helps to make a list for your "first pass" through your district, so you know what information you need to gather right off the bat so you can plan the rest of your shift. Plan to take 10 or 15 minutes per patient for a first pass, so that unless there is a huge and unexpected problem, you can see all of your patients in the first hour of your shift.

You need to check *each patient* quickly and thoroughly enough to rate them in order of acuity before you continue on. This will help you figure out who you need to consult or what you need to delegate.

## Consult or Delegate?

What if you stumble onto a problem? Patient A is desaturating and needs respiratory support or patient B's BP has tanked. How can you meet the immediate needs of one patient while still paying attention to the others?

This is where your charge nurse comes in. The first thing you need to do is make the charge nurse aware of the problem. She can call for additional assistance in the form of respiratory therapy, a house physician, or a team of people, like a rapid response team (RRT) or a medical emergency team (MET). The charge nurse can also help delegate the initial vital signs or assessment to another nurse or, most likely, ask a tech or aide to take vital signs on your other patients and report back to her. The sooner you let the charge or senior nurse know about your problem, the faster it will get solved.

## When to Wave the White Flag: Know Your Limits!

I have been a critical care nurse for 10 years, an emergency nurse for 8 years, and a clinical instructor for 5 years, and I still call for help early and often, as do many of my colleagues. I ask for help or verification in these situations:

I'm not sure if my assessment is correct.

My patient seems very different from what I got in report.

My patient is decompensating and I can't figure out why.

I've assessed and managed the patient's difficulties to the best of my knowledge, and something still doesn't seem right.

*Talk about priority setting: The priority is the patient's safety, not how smart or dumb you look.*

# How to Help the Next Shift Know the Priorities

What do you wish you had known when you started your shift? Tell that to the next shift. Alert the next nurse to these facts:

- Threats to airway, breathing, and circulation
- Trends in vital signs and urine output
- Pending treatments, tests, and results
- Responses to treatments and medications

So, how did you prioritize your care for your district based on the situation at the beginning of this chapter? Remember, we had Mr. Jones, postop and withdrawing from alcohol, Mr. Smith with a downward trending BP, Mr. Brown and his wife wondering about discharge, Ms. Green, the patient with asthma who was extubated yesterday, and the transfer from the telemetry unit who nobody's seen yet. This is how I would probably have done it:

1. I'd send a tech into the transfer from telemetry (the person I know nothing about) to take vital signs. I would have stuck my head in and eyeballed her on the way to
2. Ms. Green, the patient with asthma recently extubated (airway/breathing problem). I would have checked her mental status, respiratory rate, oxygen saturation, and lung sounds, and instructed the tech to take vitals on her while I went on to
3. Mr. Smith, whose BP is trending downward (circulation issue). I would check his pressure, heart rate, mental status, urine output. I'd check him for bleeding or other volume depletion, see if he had fluid orders, and either hang a bolus or call for MD eval (evaluation). Next stop is
4. Mr. Jones, the postop gentleman who is also withdrawing from alcohol (safety issue). He gets a mental status check, full set of vital signs, and check for postop complications like bleeding, infection, or delirium, which can all cause agitation. I'd check his CIWA (Clinical Institute Withdrawal Assessment [of Alcohol]) score, see if he needed to be medicated, and
5. Swing back through the hallway to evaluate Mr. Green and address his wife's concerns about discharge.

Total time spent would be about an hour and 15 minutes, assuming nothing was actually going badly. But now I'd have a baseline and know who I needed to check on or get vitals on more frequently, so I can continue to prioritize appropriately throughout the shift.

Ready to try it yourself?

**END-OF-CHAPTER EXERCISE: CASE STUDIES AND PRACTICE EXAMPLES**

1. Your section has eight patients (pts):

Mrs. Y, age 84, anemia, history (hx) MI (myocardial infarction), CHF, blood running

Mr. X, 28, pneumonia, looks very cachectic, bruises on his arms

Mr. B, 65, transferred to you from ICU today, s/p (status post) perforated viscous

Mr. Q, 49, transferred from G2, admitted for chest pain, has hx (history of) panic attacks

Ms. S, 33, admitted on days for exacerbation of asthma

Mrs. R, 66, CHF, COPD

Mr. G, 87, pneumonia

Mr. P, 25, transferred to you from ICU s/p multitrauma with fracture (fx) of left femur—the ICU nurse tells you he was driving while on drugs and crashed his car

   a. After taking report, which patient do you start assessing first? Why?

   b. What is the most important assessment for the majority of your patients?

   c. How often should you be making this assessment?

   d. You notice in your assessment of Mr. G that he is tachypneic and very warm. You check the flow sheet for his vital signs and find that his temperature has been WNL (within normal limits). What further information do you need in order to plan his care?

   e. Mr. P rings his bell. He's very agitated and tells you he can't breathe. He is sweaty and climbing out of the bed. What do you do?

2. It's 4 a.m. Your section of eight patients is calm. Everyone's sleeping well, no one is climbing out of bed, or screaming that they can't breathe, or telling you that they're going to call the police on you. The aide working in your section has been taking vitals signs every 4 hours, you think, but hasn't told you about any problems. Just because you have nothing else to do at the moment, you go to the bedside charts to check vitals on the patients.

a. You find that Mr. X, 75 years old, who had a high fever on days, is now 98.6°F. Do you go into the room to check him? Why or why not? What else do you need to know?

b. You find that Ms. Y, 85 years old, who is recovering from a GI bleed, has a current BP of 80/40. She has been on bedrest since she was admitted 3 days ago but had been running systolic BPs of 100 to 120. Is this significant? What do you do now?

c. Mr. Z, 35 years old and admitted for an exacerbation of asthma, has the following signs noted: BP 120/80, RR 28, temperature 99.0°F (oral), HR 120. Do you need to check on him? What will you assess?

d. Mrs. J, a 59-year-old woman s/p ORIF (open reduction and internal fixation) L hip, has the following signs documented: BP 72/38, HR 110, RR 8, temperature 96.6 °F (axillary). She is on a PCA pump. How will you assess her? What are you specifically worried about, and how will you correct the problem?

3. The charge nurse on a 36-bed unit has gone home with the flu, and now you're on your own.

- **District 1** has three "stable" patients up for discharge in the morning, one vented patient with pneumonia, one GI bleed with blood running, and two fresh postops (postoperative patients) a total of 7 patients.

- **District 2** has two patients with COPD, two GI bleeds, a R/O (rule out) TB (tuberculosis) on respiratory isolation, and three patients for discharge in the morning equaling eight patients.

- **District 3** has a withdrawing alcoholic, a patient whose BP is crashing (and there are no coronary care unit [CCU] beds), a patient on continuous bladder irrigation (CBI), an asthmatic who was extubated yesterday, and two transfers from the telemetry unit, six patients.

- District 4 has two demented patients who are s/p ORIF, a patient with CAPD (continuous abdominoperitoneal dialysis) exchanges every 4 hours, an isolation patient with methicillin-resistant *Staphylococcus aureus* (MRSA), and four patients for discharge in the morning, eight patients total.

a. How will you distribute the three aides you have?

b. The ED calls with another ethyl alcohol dependency (EtOH) withdrawal. Who gets him?

c. The nurse in District 2 is stuck in the isolation room. The aide comes to tell one of you that the GI bleed in that section has "a lot of blood" in the diaper. What do you do as a group?

d. How can you help the nurse in District 3 manage both the crashing BP and the CBI?

e. How can you help the nurse in District 4 keep the patient with CAPD from getting MRSA?

## Critical Thinking Answers

1a. Mrs. Y is elderly, has a hx of CHF, and has blood running, which can send a patient into CHF.

1b. A respiratory assessment is the most critical for the majority of these patients. CHF, asthma, pneumonia, and COPD can suddenly worsen, compromising your patient's gas exchange. Mr. P, in addition, has a long bone fracture, which predisposes him to PE (pulmonary embolism).

1c. Every 2 to 4 hours, depending on vital signs.

1d. What *antipyretics* he's been given, *how his temperature* has been taken, and what *his lungs sound* like. You'd also want to get an $O_2$ *sat*, possibly an ABG (arterial blood gas), and a chest radiograph once the resident has seen him. You should also *check his IV* (intravenous line) to make sure it's patent (he may not have gotten that last dose of antibiotics).

1e. He has a long bone fracture, which predisposes him to PE/fat embolus. Restlessness and agitation are often early signs of hypoxia, so this is not someone you want to sedate or restrain without a further assessment. Get an $O_2$ sat and a set of vital signs. Giving him ordered medication like Ativan or Valium wouldn't be terrible, as long as you continued your assessment. You should call the resident for a further evaluation. He may need a lung CT (computed tomography) or at the least some blood drawn for a d-dimer (which checks for clots).

*Remember, the restless patient needs to be evaluated, not sedated!*

2a. You need to know when he had his last dose of antibiotics and antipyretics and how his temperature was taken. It would be wise to put your hands on him and check skin temperature to correlate that with his documented temperature. You probably also want to check his BP. As patients become septic, their temperature *drops*, so a falling temperature below normal is not always good.

2b. This is a significant change. You need to check for possible causes of her drop in BP and its effect on her system. Check mental status, looking for confusion, and check urine output (these assessments evaluate perfusion of vital organs). Check her bed/diaper/bathroom for bloody stool or coffee-grounds emesis. Put $O_2$ on the patient or turn it up. Make sure she has a patent large-bore IV, and hang some normal saline because she'll need fluid resuscitation. Draw an Hemaglobin/Hematocrit (HH) and let the blood bank know you may need some blood for the patient. Have your charge nurse call the resident (and the educator) to help you.

2c. His heart rate and respiratory rate are both significantly elevated, signifying possible hypoxia. You need to check an $O_2$ sat and lung sounds. He probably needs a treatment and some supplemental oxygen.

2d. This patient is probably overmedicated. Morphine depresses the respiratory drive, resulting in the rate of 6, and causes BP to drop. The increased heart rate is compensating for both low oxygen and low perfusion. You need to shut off the PCA, administer naloxone (Narcan) as ordered, and call anesthesia to change the basal rate. Other possibilities include bleeding from the surgical site or sepsis. Get a full set of vital signs and check the patient from head to toe. Call the resident and/or education to help you.

3a. Aide 1 takes vitals on all "stable" and up-for-discharge patients every 4 hours (10 pts)

Aide 2 is assigned to take vitals and do frequent checks on the patients with dementia and the withdrawing alcoholic. He/she will also empty the Foley on the CBI patient and keep track of I/O (intake/outtake) (5-6 patients)

Aide 3 will check the GI bleeds and the fresh postops (5-6 patients)

3b. District 3 or 4 because there's an aide already assigned to keep an eye on those patients.

3c. The nurse in District 4 can check on this patient, leaving the other two nurses to keep an eye on the other patient and/or call for medical backup if there is indeed a problem. You'll need to make sure that patient has a patent IV because the patient may need fluids and/or blood. Call for backup sooner rather than later.

3d. The aide assigned can keep track of the Foley. The patient with the crashing BP should have an RRT (Rapid Response Team), a clinical supervisor, or a house physician at the bedside to manage their care, to allow the nurse to at least direct the care of her other patients,

3e. Someone from District 1 or 3, who has no isolation patients, would be the best choice. Looks like tonight is a group nursing night.

# [CHAPTER 5]

# Patient Safety

ELIZABETH A. HENNEMAN

$P$atient safety has always been a priority for nurses. Florence Nightingale was one of the first nurse leaders to recognize that much of the work that nurses do is to protect patients against potential hazards that occur in the hospital setting (Nightingale, 1969). But only recently have health-care professionals and the public come to recognize just how many hazards exist in our health-care settings or, more importantly, the pivotal role that nurses play in keeping patients safe.

Many of the first lessons we learn in nursing school are related to patient safety. Examples include proper handwashing, the "six rights" of medication administration, the importance of effective communication, and keeping a patient's side rails up when the patient is confused or sedated.

In 2000, the Institute of Medicine (IOM) published a report called "To Err Is Human." In this report, the IOM suggested that up to 98,000 patients in the United States die each year from medical error (Kohn, Corrigan, & Donaldson, 2000). This number of deaths is greater than the number of patients in the United States who die each year from automobile accidents, AIDS, or breast cancer. This first IOM publication was a clear "call to action" to the health-care community to examine our practice and improve health-care safety.

Nurses play a critical role in patient safety. In our role as 24-hour frontline providers, nurses are well positioned to identify patient safety risks and implement strategies to keep patients safe. Students and new nurses are often overwhelmed at the responsibility they have for keeping patients safe. I'm still overwhelmed, and I've been a nurse for 30 years!

*I had no idea how important nurses were in patient safety. I have come to realize that they are the final safety valve for so many things. (John)*

*I wasn't surprised to discover that nurses played such a large role in maintaining patient safety. However, I didn't realize that maintaining patient safety would require nurses to have an extensive knowledge of pharmacology. Medications have become such a huge part of how we treat people in this country, and it is the nurse's responsibility to manage all of the different medications and make sure nothing goes wrong. To do this, nurses must be familiar with how different drugs interact and issues pertaining to allergies and cross-reactivity of the drugs. (Student)*

*I realized going into nursing that there would be a lot of responsibility. But I didn't realize how truly everything you do could pretty much have an adverse effect if done poorly or incorrectly. (Anna)*

*I didn't realize the responsibility the nurse takes on each day. I work in peds, so general safety is a constant concern [i.e., fall prevention, keeping an eye on kids when parents step out/are absent, making sure to remove all trash (I'm always afraid a baby will swallow syringe caps or other small objects).] (Abigail)*

*I feel as though most of what has been emphasized in school about patient safety pertains to safe medication administration and infection control. The importance of handwashing is emphasized more than any other patient safety measure. In every class it seems as though the professor makes a point to reiterate the fact that handwashing is the best thing we can do as nurses to prevent infection and keep our patients safe. Medication checks are another way that we have been taught to keep our patients safe. I will follow the six rights of medication administration before giving meds, which includes confirming the patient's identity before giving a med and checking the med against the patient's medication administration record (MAR) when it comes out of the drawer, before I give it to the patient and after the patient has taken it. Checking allergies and knowing how different drugs interact will also help to keep patients safe. (Student)*

# I'M SO WORRIED I'LL MAKE A MISTAKE!

Anxiety about making mistakes is common in concern of student nurses, new graduates, and experienced nurses alike. All nurses make mistakes.

Personally, I worry the most about the nurse who says, "I never have and never will make a mistake." Nurses are human, and therefore it is inevitable that they will make a mistake at some point.

Nurses who say they have never made a mistake are most likely unaware that their actions were in error because their mistakes caused no immediate negative effects. The smartest nurses recognize that they *could* make a mistake and do the best they can to prevent it. And the best nurses report their mistakes so we all can learn how to do things better.

One of the lessons taught by the IOM report "To Err Is Human" was that there are two main categories of error. The first is called human error. This type of error is less common but still to be expected whenever human beings are involved in a process. And because of the nature of our work as nurses, there is a lot of human interaction, so we can expect human error.

The second, more common type of error is called system error. System errors are created by organizational cultures, administrative decisions, and technical issues that alone or in combination impact patient care. For example, if a hospital has decided to use a computerized order entry system that generates a medication list and then results in the distribution of medications before the nurse has a chance to review the patient's medication history and allergies with the patient, there is a greater chance an error may be made.

One of our most serious safety issues is the lack of evidence-based practices (as opposed to "doing things the way we have always done them").

*It's confusing how it seems like every nurse has a different way of doing things. Sure there are best practices, but it seems like there are just so many ways to do anything, without a clear best way. (Anna)*

Despite our knowledge of the extent of system issues that lead to error, many nurses, including novices, tend to focus on human error. This is largely because they want to "do it right" and not make a mistake (especially in front of the instructor!). It usually takes students and novice nurses a while to start to "see" the system issues that may negatively affect their ability to give safe care. However, the "fresh eyes" of the new nurses are often clearer in seeing system problems and the reality of a way of working that may not be optimal.

John, a student nurse, tells the story of how his first injection didn't go as smoothly as planned.

*I wanted to share my error experience. Or at least I feel it was an error. I was scared (about giving an injection) but tried to convey confidence. I drew up the med correctly and was going with my clinical instructor to the patient's room and I started to sweat, not just a little but a bucket.*

*I found the appropriate site, and gave a darting motion (that any dart-throwing man would have envied). I didn't let go of the needle but instead slammed it into the patient. The patient's nurse said, "Great mother of God!" (or something to that effect). By this time I was an emotional wreck.*

*The rest of that evening, everyone, peers and staff, proceeded to make fun of me and give me a general hard time (in fun most of the time). The patient did survive but had a nice big bruise on her belly as proof of my excessive darting motion. Needless to say, the next clinical day, my instructor had me giving two injections. I did them nearly perfectly. Man, I was nervous, and everyone was milling outside the room to see how I did. Thank God I figured it out.*

The type of error John describes is a human error. The three types of human errors are skill based, rule based, and knowledge based. Of the three, it is logical to expect students and new graduates to recognize skill-based errors (or at least acknowledge their lack of skill). However, rule-based and knowledge-based errors are also common and occur with both novice and experienced nurses.

# WHAT ARE THE MOST COMMON ERRORS?

The most common errors in health care are related to the failure to communicate properly. Communication failures typically fall under the category of system errors (as opposed to human error). Communication failures can occur between any and all members of the health-care team, such as between two nurses, a nurse and physician, a nurse and patient, and so on. For example, if the off-going nurse giving report to the oncoming nurse does not have access to all pertinent patient history information because of a delay in accessing medical records, a communication error could occur because the system does not support the nurse's ability to give a comprehensive report.

Keeping open lines of communication between yourself and all members of the team, especially the patient and family, is critical to providing safe care. When the Joint Commission on Accreditation of Healthcare Organizations (JCAHO) reports on serious adverse events (called sentinel events), they almost always report on the existence of gaps in the communication process.

One common misconception is that the most important type of communication needed for patient safety is between nurses and nurses or nurses and physicians. This is not correct. Communicating with the patient and family is probably the most important communication to providing safe care. If the patient and family are not actively involved in providing information and in the decision-making process, it is highly likely that patient safety will be placed in jeopardy. Some of these safety issues may not be evident during the hospitalization period but may occur only after the patient has been discharged. For example, the failure to include family members of the patients in the teaching regarding their medications may result in a drug overdose or the failure to take necessary medications.

In addition, communication with other members of the health-care team, such as respiratory therapists, physical therapists, technical assistants, and nurse's aides, is imperative for providing safe, efficient, and effective care.

The following scenario described by Kathie gives an example of why communication with the family is so important.

*The patient had just returned from an MRI and had a lot of family around, and then they left. The patient's bed alarm was off and she never used the call bell for assistance. She got out of bed by herself and fell. She hit the metal sink cabinet between the two beds, adjacent to the bathroom, so her elbow was bleeding and the hematoma on her lower back was huge and she also became incontinent. There had not been a fall on the shifts that I've worked, but I realize now how quickly they can happen and how serious the consequences are. So I will not forget to keep the side rails up and bed alarms on!*

This is an example of what could happen when there is a gap in communication between the nurse and the family. The family should have been alerted to notify the nurse when they were leaving so that the side rails could be placed in an upright position.

# WHAT CAN I DO TO KEEP MY PATIENTS SAFE?

Research suggests that experienced nurses use certain strategies to keep their patients safe (Henneman & Gawlinski, 2004) and to recover (identify, interrupt, and correct errors when they occur). These strategies include teamwork, anticipation, surveillance, and double-checking.

## Teamwork

You will *never* be able to care for a patient all by yourself. It doesn't matter how many years you've been a nurse. It always takes a team. The "team" is composed of the patient, his or her family, and other health-care providers. Other team personnel besides the patient and family depends on the situation. For example, for many hospitalized patients, the respiratory or physical therapist plays a critical role in providing care.

One of the reasons teamwork is so important is because it promotes communication. As mentioned earlier, communication errors are the number one source of errors in health care. The failure to communicate important information is a significant source of error. And remember, communication with the patient and family may be the *most* important communication you engage in.

Some basic communication strategies are those related to patient and provider identification. For example, it is critical that you confirm your patient's identity by asking your patient to state their first and last name and date of birth. It is also important to verify that the information on the identification (ID) band matches the information provided by the patient and the information on the treatment plan or medication. New technologies, such as bar coding are useful in making this process safer.

## Anticipation

The ability to anticipate a patient's potential risk for harm is very important. It is a skill developed over time. One strategy to learn this skill is to discuss with instructors, preceptors, or experienced nurses the high-risk problems that you may expect to experience when caring for a particular patient.

Jonathan, a nurse with several years of experience, describes an event when the failure to anticipate harm (because of system issues), resulted in a poor outcome for a patient.

*I do a routine check of the telemetry station and ask the nurse how long Bed 22 has been in rapid a-fib? The nurse tells me that they have tried lopressor push, then diltiazem push, but nothing has worked, and now the patient's blood pressure is compromised, hanging on at 85/55. I ask if the ICU team has been involved. They just look at me and say. "You have no idea what this night was like!" The unfortunate thing is that room 22 coded at 0705. If more emphasis had been placed on getting the unit to look at her, she may have been in the unit at 0400. Now we are shocking her heart at 0715 because she is in v-fib. She does not convert, and she becomes asystolic. At 0732 she is pronounced, and every nurse in the room has a look of disbelief.*

*I am the permanent charge nurse on a medical telemetry floor at a well-respected hospital. This is not an uncommon event for me to walk into at the start of my shift. More often than not, there are simply not enough resources on nights to combat situations like these.*

*I've noticed over time as a student in the hospital that desensitization occurs and a casual approach can develop. (John)*

## Surveillance

Surveillance, as it relates to promoting and maintaining patient safety, is defined as the purposeful, ongoing collection and analysis of information about patients and their environment (McCloskey-Dochterman & Bulechek, 2004). It differs from the traditional concept of monitoring in that it is specifically directed at a patient and family's unique situation and needs.

Sarah describes how surveillance played a role in her appreciation of the risk her patient faced as she recovered in the hospital.

*On my first day of clinical, an independent and active 90-year old woman was admitted to the med-surg floor for dehydration and other debilitating effects of the flu. As I helped her get settled in, I felt keenly aware of the risk she faced from a nosocomial infection as she recovered from her illness in the hospital. Minimizing the spread of infection was a consideration of mine before I started nursing school. I'll play in the dirt, and kiss dogs and kids, but I'm conscious about the transfer of infection in public places. During my first semester in nursing school, I discovered that this consciousness was an asset to me in the hospital rather than an incapacitating force or hindrance.*

Surveillance includes not only recognizing the patient's potential for risk but also "knowing the patient." This concept of "knowing the patient" is increasingly being recognized as integral for improving patient outcomes. Knowing the patient includes having an understanding of the patient's past experiences and his or her responses to treatment (Tanner, Benner, Chesla, & Gordon, 1993; Whittemore, 2000).

Surveillance also involves paying close attention to these risks and ensuring the environment is ready should something happen. Rachel describes a situation where surveillance, knowing the patient, and attending to the family, played a role in patient safety.

*I was assigned a patient who had been admitted to the hospital with a diagnosis of encephalitis of unknown origin. She had had two seizures before arriving at this particular hospital and another three seizures after being admitted. I met her on a Tuesday, and aside from being incredibly energetic she was like most other 6-year-olds. Several days after I cared for her, my patient had another seizure and was transferred to the ICU.*

*Wednesday was seeming to be a good day, I took her vitals, did my assessment, and again we played games. This time I noticed though that she was not accommodating with her eyes as she should when I tested PERRLA. I let the nurse know and continued to check her neurologic function for the rest of the day. At about 1730, I started having a conversation with her parents about their hometown and their other daughter. Twenty minutes into the conversation, my patient became unresponsive. Her mom recognized this as a seizure, and we immediately hit the call button and yelled down the hallway and a team of nurses came running.*

The moral of the story is (1) Always do a through assessment (i.e., PERRLA, check and recheck, and monitor) and (2) Always make sure to check the room for all of the equipment that may be necessary in case of an emergency.

# Double-Checking

One of my favorite sayings in my roles as a nursing instructor, clinical nurse specialist, and preceptor has always been "check, check, double-check." Both novice and expert nurses agree that double-checking is critical to ensuring patient safety. In many instances, double-checking is defined as the nurses themselves "reconfirming" that they are administering the correct treatment (e.g., looking at the name of the medication on the package and then looking a second time). Other types of double-checking involve one nurse asking another nurse or physician to confirm that they are making the correct decision.

John tells of his experience in a neonatal intensive care unit (NICU) when the nurse he was working with double-checked the amount of medication that had been ordered by the physician.

*Just yesterday, I was on an NICU and a resident physician wrote an order for a newborn to get glucose for hypoglycemia. In writing the order the resident misplaced the decimal point and ordered 10 times the normal dose, which would have jumped this newborn's blood sugar way too high. Who knows what problems it would have caused? But the nurse I was observing checked the order, checked the mg/kg calculation, and discovered the error. She immediately informed the physician, who thanked her and wrote a new order for the correct amount. I then witnessed the nurse check the order and the math again, just to be sure. I was impressed and glad the nurse made the catch. I understand why we check the orders and check the meds. Med safety is very important.*

Abigail reinforced the importance of double-checking.

*Double-check everything! Ask questions even if you think it's stupid. Rely on senior staff. Write things down. Check blood products, lab labels, and chemo at the bedside. Double-check med dosing.*

# FUTURE DIRECTIONS: THOUGHTS FROM STUDENTS AND PRACTICING NURSES

*How to make a hospital safer? Beyond education and implementation of standards, a safer hospital might be built from the ground up, with an environment created by architects with a focus on human nature and efficient space. I think team building among health-care workers would also improve safety in the hospital; given the time and incentive to communicate and work together, a health-care team could be higher functioning and self-monitoring. I would want to place my own care in the hands of a team of people who have been given the incentive, time, and tools to work together in the hospital environment. (Anna)*

*I think there should be longer/more formal mentorship programs in health care (not just nursing). As novices, there are many situations when I fear my lack of experience could be dangerous to a patient. No patient should have poor care secondary to simple inexperience. If nurses were trained more on a one-on-one basis with more supervision and on-the-job teaching, I think patient safety would benefit. (Anna)*

*The gap between the clinical setting and the classroom setting is disconcerting to me. There is a complacency in the hospital that breeds error, which may have to do with the high patient load, lack of continuity in personnel and/or patients, and the fact that when mistakes are made, the people making the errors often never see the consequences. (Anna)*

# SOME FINAL THOUGHTS AND ADVICE FROM NURSES ON SAFETY

*We are the eyes and ears for the MDs. A good nurse is key to patient safety, no matter how small the concern. (Abigail)*

*If you get into good habits now, you will be set for your career. (Laura)*

*I think the best way to keep patients safe is to assess my own strength and weaknesses. By knowing what I can and cannot do, I am able to find ways to either (1) improve myself in providing safe care or (2) know when to ask for help from other students, nurses, and instructors. (Angela)*

# ASK YOURSELF THESE QUESTIONS

Regardless of where you are in your career as a nurse, a student, new graduate, or experienced nurse, you should prepare yourself to work in challenging situations where there will be many situations when you will need help in order to prevent errors and keep patients safe. Here are some questions you should think about:

1. What are my own strengths and weaknesses?
2. Who can I trust/go to when I have a question? Who will I feel safe with?
3. What are "system" issues that need to be addressed to give safe care?
4. What is the process used in our setting to address these issues?

# References

Henneman, E., & Gawlinski, A. (2004). A near-miss model for describing the nurse's role in the recovery of medical errors. *Journal of Professional Nursing, 20,* 196–201.

Kohn, L. T., Corrigan, M., & Donaldson, M. S., eds.; Committee on Quality of Health Care in America; Institute of Medicine. (2000). *To Err is Human: Building a Safer Health System.* Washington, DC: National Academy Press.

McCloskey-Dochterman, J. M., & Bulechek, G. M., eds. (2004). Surveillance: Safety. In: *Nursing Interventions Classification* (4th ed.). St. Louis, MO: Mosby Year Book.

Nightingale, F. (1969). *Notes on Nursing.* NY: Dover Publications.

Tanner, C. A., Benner, P., Chesla, C., & Gordon, D. R. (1993). The phenomenology of knowing the patient. *Image: Journal of Nursing Scholarship, 25,* 273–280.

Whittemore, R. (2000). Consequences of not "knowing the patient." *Clinical Nurse Specialist, 14,* 75–81.

# [CHAPTER 6]

# Bonding

*There is no house like the house of belonging*

—David White

**W**hen you feel a bond with someone, there is a chemistry, a connection. When you find the right place to work that fits who you are, there is a gut feeling, instantly, like a blink, that makes you feel like "this is the place for me!" Malcolm Gladwell, the author of *Blink* (2005) describes that instantaneous connection we have or do not have with each other. If you are wondering, "How do I know if this is the right job for me?" the answer is that you need to feel that instant connection. You need to feel like you belong there. When was the last time you felt that connection when you first met someone? Who was it? You know that feeling. Pay attention:

1. What was your response when you contacted the organization where you think you'd like to work?
2. Did you like the human resource person?
3. What sense did you get when you spoke to the nurse manager? The manager is a key player in your future.

Your body will tell you if the situation feels right. Listen. When I was a staff nurse I could tell if I was going to have a good shift, not by who the patients were but by what staff I was working with. I learned this in my first nursing position at a prestigious New England hospital. At 22 years old, I recognized the critical effect that the nurses I worked with had on my ability to function in my role as staff nurse.

*I'd unlock the big wooden doors to the unit, walk across the main entryway to the glassed-in nurses' station, unlock the door, and look at the sheet taped to the window. Once I saw who was on the shift with me, I'd either let out a sigh of relief and proceed into report with a smile or tense up with a sense of reserve and take shift report thinking, "How are we going to get through the next 8 hours?" It's no surprise patients would stick their head over the half door to get a peek at who was working next and announce to the other patients draped over the well-worn couches in the vestibule, "Oh, this will be a good evening" or "Oh no, might as well give me some meds now because I am going to have a rough night!" The patients knew as well as I did that the tenor of the shift depended on who was working together.*

"There is no house like the house of belonging," the last line of David Whyte's poem, says it all (p. 6, 1997). Whyte recognized how critical it is to feel like you are connected with others, and this could not be more true for the new nurse who enters her or his first position. From the *First Year Study* we know that the new nurse needs to feel recognized and valued as a part of the unit staff. Feeling like you are welcomed by the other nurses and a valued participant on the team of health-care providers is key to your success in your new job. A sense of belonging enables the new nurse to feel comfortable enough to learn and valued enough to ask questions. As a new nurse you need to be able to depend on your peers so you can be independent enough to give patient care. Belonging can make the difference between staying in a position or counting the days until you can look for a new one.

You want to make the right career decision for yourself. I know when you are looking for a job you will get all wrapped up in how you come across, thinking, "Do I know enough? Will they like me? Will they offer me the job?" And, yes, it is important to be prepared, but take a moment to check in and see how you are feeling about the people you are meeting. Do they make you feel welcome, like you belong there?

## FEELING LIKE ONE OF THE GANG

As the new nurse you need to feel welcomed, accepted, and an important member of the team. Nursing is not a "me" job; it is the "we" approach that works. You cannot provide nursing alone. Although you are assigned to your own patients, it takes a team to provide the care. You need a whole backup staff to assist each other so you can give the level of care your patient deserves. Be aware of the importance of good working relationships. Pay attention to the feeling you get from the first time you make a job contact.

1. When you call or e-mail to learn about a position, are you responded to in a warm, welcoming way or do you already feel like a number? That tells you something about the institution you may be working for.

2. Does the human resource person get back to you in a timely fashion?

3. When you were interviewed, did you feel like you were being grilled or having a comfortable conversation?

4. When you asked for the interviewer to describe the staff on the unit, what was her response?

5. Look up the mission and philosophy of the organization. That tells you about what they value.

    a. Does teaching come first?

    b. Where is the patient in the philosophy?

    c. Do your values fit with the hospitals?

    d. What is the nursing philosophy?

    e. Does that fit with your ideals?

In the *First Year Study*, a group of new nurses whom I met with were second bachelor new grads who all worked in different facilities and in different specialty areas. One new grad was on labor and delivery nights, one was on telemetry nights, and the other was on the day shift in the Emergency Department. As students, these three nurses were at the top of their class and were invested in becoming well-respected, competent nurses. When I opened the interview with, "So what is the first year like?" all three answered, "If it weren't for the other nurses, I don't know what I'd do." Tammi observed,

*On labor and delivery at night, it can be a very busy place. No birth is ever the same. The other nurses are so helpful. They always check in with me and make sure I am doing okay.*

"I know," Michaela from the ER chimed in. "*They encourage me to ask questions. It is clear to me I'd never be able to function at this level so soon and at this fast pace if it wasn't for the other nurses. They are there when I need them. I know they want me to succeed.*"

It is important to get the sense that the team you are working with wants you to succeed, not just the supervisor or your preceptor but that everyone is pitching in and rooting for you to be successful in your first position.

Once Tammi, Micheala, and Maria described the camaraderie that they each felt from the other nurses, it was telling to hear that each one of them, although not on their preferred shift, liked their job. All three new grads felt part of their unit. They all felt they had a bond with the more experienced nurses, there was an esprit de corps, and they were in this together.

A relationship that is based on shared interests, feelings, or experiences can lead to the sense of bonding. One of the three outcomes from the *First Year Study* was that the sense of bonding with your peer group was essential for making it in your first position. Considering the high first-year attrition rate, it is worth it for both you and the organization to feel like you have the support you need to be a success. Liz suggests,

*You have to figure out who can help you out. It is like being new at college. You have to reach out and make new relationships. You have to come in with an open mind and make relationships with all the staff. I try to help others out so they will be there for me.*

Many new nurses echo this idea: "Look to offer to help others so they will help you and you will be seen as a team player." Being flexible with the needs of your patients and peers is a way to win team members over. Once you offer to help others, when you need assistance or to change your schedule, your new colleagues are more likely to help out. A recently hired nurse accepted a position in a magnet hospital that had a new grad residency program. Sarah enthusiastically exclaimed, "From the interview on, I felt like I was being recruited and they wanted me." Sarah said she felt a bond with the three nurse managers that came to the group interview. You should expect to feel like Sarah, welcomed and encouraged. The new grads who liked their jobs felt encouraged from the interview on. The facilities that attracted new grads put out a warm welcome, offered support up front, and let them know they understood what it was like to be a new nurse.

In those first contacts you want to look at how they select new employees. Does the human resources department decide on the unit where you should have an interview? Do the nurse managers have a say in where the new nurse fits? The hiring and selection process differs in each facility. In one hospital, the nurse recruiter chooses who goes to the units that have openings. In another hospital, the nurse managers who need new staff members interview the new recruits in a group, describing their units and giving the new grads an opportunity to consider which unit would fit best with their interests. Don't be shy in asking about the hiring process so you can be prepared for the next level of interviewing. One recent grad was asked to work a shift as part of the two-day interview process that began with a standard interview and ended with shadowing a nurse for a day. This is an ideal approach for the floor to get to know you and for you to get to know the floor before you sign on.

During the interview ask for the details of the orientation. Is there

1. A clear, organized plan for orientation?

2. A focus on your experience coming into a new system, *or* is it the usual emphasis on the organization and you figuring out a way to adapt to their needs? There is an important difference here; look for it.

3. A guaranteed preceptor program? Be careful with the approach of starting out in orientation and by the second week they need staff so all of a sudden you are pulled on the floor full time. This may feel like you are so good you can skip right over orientation, but in the long run you are doing yourself a disservice not to insist that you gradually move into the staff role.

4. Ongoing educational, social, and emotional structured supports throughout the first year? Ask:

   a. Are there ongoing educational offerings for new grads?

   b. Is there a planned social time with other new grads and preceptors?

   c. Is there a planned time for new grads to process their emotions? A time to process the experience of being so new, share the fear of making a mistake, or reflect on the grief over your first death?

5. The bottom line is, does the orientation look more like school, 6 hours of classes? Or does it look interesting and inviting? The orientation should help you get acclimated, review skills, and build your confidence.

Research has demonstrated that new grads going into today's complex health-care system need substantial support, the right information, extra resources, and a variety of opportunities so they can provide the best care, keep patients safe, and develop their critical thinking skills. We know nurses feel empowered when they get the information, opportunities, resources, and support they need (Chandler, 1991). As the low person on the totem pole, feeling empowered is not a bad idea. In the *First Year Study*, good relationships was the most important variable to new nurses' success. In Roche, Morsi, & Chandler's (2009) recent study of nurse experts, the information, resources, and opportunities had an influence on the relationships with peers and expert nurses were empowering, then the nurse was able to move from being proficient to being an expert. Relationships or bonding with your coworkers is the first requirement for making it as a new nurse. Orientation should provide you with opportunities to connect with other new grads, discover facility resources, and experience focused learning. In Sarah's first job she reports, "There was no pressure to know everything right away." She described an orientation that focused on managing your stress and your anxiety. On the first day the orientation leaders told us "We don't expect anything from you today, tomorrow, or next week. Just try to show up on time." Sarah said, "Nobody expects you to know ANYTHING . . . No really! Anything you do know is a bonus. Somebody told me this on my first day, and it made a world of difference in how I felt." That is the key: How do you feel? To learn you need a safe environment balanced with excitement, energy and a relaxed, open attitude.

There is an exciting development for new grads in acute care facilities you should know about: the new nurse residency program designed to complement the orientation experience. Acute care facilities have finally recognized that new grads enter nursing with some book knowledge and a brief survey of clinical experience, but when just starting out, considering today's complexity and acuity of patient care, all new nurses need extended, structured support. Traditionally, new grads were expected to hit the ground running, but today's challenging acute care environment has required both education and hospitals to rethink the model of the month-long orientation and then you are on your own. As Sarah recognized,

*Nursing school is like planting seeds of knowledge. When you graduate, all you have is a pile of seeds. GREAT! What are you gonna do with that? It isn't until you begin working and giving those seeds what they need to grow that your knowledge comes to fruition.*

Residency programs are designed to nurture what new grads bring to the job by providing an environment for the new nurse to flourish. Even if you will not be working in a facility with a residency program, it is important to know that the evidence shows multiple layers of support are essential for new nurses. If you know what is offered to new residents, you'll know what it takes to survive and thrive. By being aware of what residency programs offer the new nurse, you can suggest some supports for your new position.

# RESIDENCY PROGRAMS: WHAT ARE THEY?

Residency programs are often year-long structured programs designed to:

- Teach new graduates clinical skills
- Expand on analytic thinking
- Develop a reflective practice
- Foster the new nurse's contribution to improve practice
- Provide emotional support
- Create a career advancement plan (Nurse Executive Center, 2006)

New grads who have had the opportunity to participate in a residency program report their experience was outstanding! From my review of residency programs and new grads' experience, I believe residency programs provide the level of support and guidance all new grads should have. Acute care facilities developed extended residency programs in the recognition that new graduates need assistance negotiating the complex healthcare system, learning how to manage shift work and providing care for several acutely ill patients. Although each facility creates a program to meet the needs of their organization, these are some common characteristics of residency programs:

- They are designed as a transition from school to practice
- They help new grads right out of nursing school
- They include all new grads to create a supportive peer group
- They emphasize critical thinking

Do you think a residency program would be right for you? If so, you need to look for a hospital that has a program and ask questions about the goals of the residency program to see if it will fit your needs. The seven primary goals of exemplary programs are as follows:

1. Bridge gaps in a new graduate's skill set and organizational expectations.
2. Connect the book knowledge of school to real-life clinical challenges.
3. Ensure consistent support from leadership and peers.
4. Foster an espirit de corps among residents.
5. Increase residents' understanding of the health-care system.

6. Empower new nurses to contribute to the improvement of practice.

7. Demonstrate opportunities for professional growth (Nursing Executive Center, 2006).

- *Bridge gaps in a new graduate's skill set and organizational expectations.* The curriculum in the residency programs provides a supportive, nonthreatening environment while the new nurse is learning about complex areas of nursing care such as pain management, palliative care, skin care, or SBAR (Situation-Background-Assessment-Recommendation) communication. The program meetings provide a safe place to ask questions and an opportunity to learn from peers on the same level. Case examples are developed from the experience the new nurse has on the unit. Participants are encouraged to write clinical narratives about their current experiences with patients and staff so that the classes are new nurse-centered rather than instructor driven. The nurse residents are invited to identify topics so that the class facilitators can invite experts to explain their areas of practice. Simulation labs are widely used to practice patient assessment and team communication with the belief that practicing on a patient simulator provides a safe bridge between school-book knowledge and in-person clinical practice.

- *Connect the book knowledge of school to real-life clinical challenges.* Case studies using critical thinking and reflective practice are learning opportunities provided at the new nurse seminar so the generalizations of book knowledge can be applied to the individual subtleties of practice. For example, the book instructions for a catheterization looks like you learn how to maintain a sterile field and follow the steps for the procedure and you're good! That is, until you walk in and find the patient is obese, with dementia, and too frightened to relax and cooperate. This is where a conversation with experts and peers is invaluable. In addition to real-life case studies, programs use video clips of practice situations so the new nurse can participate in unit-based activities that strengthen skills demonstrated in the video. Reflective journaling is a valuable learning approach used to capture the individual nurse's response to new knowledge and share with other nurse residents. Group cohesion develops from sharing insights and receiving feedback (Nurse Executive Center, 2006, p. 16).

- *Ensure consistent support from leadership and peers.* Being a nurse looked good on *ER* and *Scrubs,* but now it is time for a full work week, multiple shifts, and weekends with no faculty hovering nearby. Although the faculty, clinical rotations, or your patient assignment while you were in school may not have been perfect; you always had faculty supervision and backup, worked just a couple of shifts a week, and had a limited patient load. Now you are expected to work three 12-hour shifts, function from 7 a.m. to 7 p.m. and work weekends and major holidays all without your school support network. Residency programs recognize the dramatic shift from school to work and have developed a variety of support mechanisms, for example, clinical coaches that are hand-picked expert nurses who may be on the same unit or on a different unit or may even be in a different facility. In the Wisconsin Nurse Residency Program, the coaches receive education on supporting new graduates, developing reflective skills, and providing a monthly meeting with residents to discuss successes and challenges (Nurse Executive Center, 2006, p. 18). Facilitator-led, resident-focused reflection circles occur once a month to meet with other new nurses and share practice concerns and challenges. In the Children's Memorial Hospital program, the bimonthly transition group is led by a nurse or a social worker, or the chaplain, to give nurses the opportunity to discuss topics they have identified, such as working as a team, communicating with physicians, or managing conflict (Nurse Executive Center, 2006, p. 19). The groups are designed to provide opportunities every nurse needs: develop networks with peers, foster coping strategies, and provide time for reflection. If you do not have a residency program, you need to look for opportunities to build these key factors into your first year of practice.

- *Foster an esprit de corps among residents.* New grads, although this feels like the most important year of their life, can get lost in the busyness of hospital activities. They blend in or are seen as just one more job for the already burdened staff. Residency programs were designed to keep the focus on the new grad experience, celebrate accomplishments, and be recognized in formal ceremonies. Whether formal or informal, make sure you have regular feedback on your accomplishments. Being new on any unit may feel isolating, disconnecting, and overwhelming. It is important to be able to find like-minded souls. The University of New Mexico Hospital program designed a uniform for the residents so they could recognize each other and are known by nurse and physician colleagues (Nurse Executive Center, 2006, p. 20). Another program created a physical space with a conference room and lounge just for new nurses. Peer connections were encouraged at work and after hours.

- *Increase residents' understanding of the health-care system.* Our federal government and all of its experts cannot figure out the health-care system, so how can a new grad? Nurses are at the hub of patient care and are expected to know what resources to call on for their patients and assist their patients in negotiating the system. That is a big job. The Yale New Haven residency program offers a course on the health-care system to assist the new grad in understanding how accreditation affects their position, what other departments have available to patients, and how to understand health policy (Nurse Executive Center, 2006, p. 22). The All Children's Hospital program has residents spend a day on units that their unit receives referrals from or refer to, such as the OR (operating room) and the PACU (postanesthesia care unit). The resident then has the opportunity to learn where the patient is going or what the patient has experienced prior to coming to their unit. The program reports that "looping" of patient care is to help residents to understand the continuum of care, the role of their colleagues on their referral units, and the experience of patients and families being transferred from one unit to another. A goal is to develop relationships with nurses on other units to improve the quality and the continuity of care (Nurse Executive Center, 2006, p. 23).

- *Empower new nurses to contribute to the improvement of practice.* New grads bring new eyes to the practice environment. As a nurse manager, I would purposely hire two new grads a year and encourage them to question the usual routine and volunteer to participate in practice committees so we could have a fresh perspective on an old issue. As a college professor I hear students come up with keen observations of taken-for-granted practice and propose unique solutions to nagging problems. Several residency programs recognize the potential of their new grads and encourage them to participate in committees, research projects, and root cause analysis.

- *Demonstrate opportunities for professional growth.* As a nurse manager, from the first interview I would ask new nurses what they envisioned their next step was and what they had in mind for their long-term career plan. Many had not thought beyond the job they were interviewing for, so this question helped them look toward their future. Inquiring about their next career step also communicated that I was interested in them as individuals and not just trying to fill a vacant position. My philosophy was that if I supported the new nurses' growth and development, they would be more likely to stay longer. This approach worked well even for those who had a plan to return to school in the not too distant future. I supported their educational pursuits by helping them to figure out practice experiences that would make them more attractive candidates for graduate school. Then when they were accepted into programs, the nurses felt such an allegiance to our unit that they came back to work per diem, which increased staff cohesiveness and continuity of patient care.

The residency programs provide the support and connections new grads need. In hospitals that do not have formal programs, preceptors are looked to as coaches and confidants.

## THE PRECEPTOR RELATIONSHIP IS KEY

The new nurses we spoke with reinforced the importance of the preceptor relationship. Whether the preceptor fits with the new grad or not, the experience can still provide a learning opportunity.

Maria comments,

*The people who are going to be your teachers/preceptors have a great role in whether or not you feel successful. I had two very different experiences. I oriented on the day shift for 3 months. My preceptors during this time were phenomenal—constantly challenging my critical thinking skills, allowing me space to figure things out on my own, but stepping in when I needed it. They offered constant positive reinforcement. This type of relationship made me more eager to learn and it slowly helped to build my self-confidence.*

*Then I went to orient on nights for a couple of weeks before I was on my own. My preceptor on nights did not talk to me—literally. In fact she was very intimidating and kind of scary. My stomach used to hurt every time I worked during that time. I was afraid to ask her things for fear that she would think I was a complete idiot. But what I did do was figure out who the other resources were on my unit— the other nurses. I also learned how to look a lot of things up—policies, information about conditions that my patients were coming in with (which I'd never heard of). It bothered me for a long time that she was like this with me, but eventually I got over it . . . and so did she. In those torturous weeks I learned a lot about myself and my ability to be able to figure things out. I have worked with this woman for over a year now, and just last week she said "nice job" to me for the very first time.*

*I guess my point is that you are not always going to be paired up with someone who is as nurturing as you'd like. But as miserable as I felt, I was still learning and I continued to remind myself that this was not about her. It was about me figuring things out.*

This is an important message from Maria as she reflects back after a year out of school. You can expect a preceptor to be challenging, letting the new grad figure it out, yet stepping in when you need.

After a year in practice, Demetri reflected back on his preceptor experience,

*During senior year I had a terrific internship; my preceptor was just right for me. There was chemistry between us. She was the preceptor I needed at that time to build confidence in myself. She had a therapeutic way, understood how to act and react, was compassionate, and a good role model. Wonderful, really amazing.*

*When I was hired into the same facility, in the orientation I was paired with someone else as a preceptor. She was not as warm and fuzzy but really hit me over the head with skills. I feel like the unit went out of the way to cultivate my practice. The whole unit was behind my success, not my preceptor alone.*

Demetri offers some insight into the learning process,

*I felt it was a challenge to build myself up to have more than two patients. I had to get up to four. I really didn't get enough empirical practice in school or learn how to talk to the physician. Though I had a 320-hour internship, I still did not know what resources to call when. And when I started I needed my preceptor glued to me.*

A new grad recognizes,

*Preceptors come in all shapes and sizes, or more accurately all ages and personalities. Some new nurses recommend the senior, experienced nurse; others say the nurse who is just a couple years out can relate to being new and has a better understanding about how to teach. My preceptors have been the most important people in my professional development. I had both types of preceptors: the young but gentle guide and as I termed the second, "the benevolent drill sergeant."*

Another new grad recalls,

*I had the same preceptor pretty much the whole time. I basically followed her around for 2 weeks. And didn't really do anything. Then she gave me one patient; then she gave me two patients. Eventually I had all of her patients. I was with her for 6 weeks; which was sort of up for negotiation if I felt like I needed more time. The supervisor would check in with me. "OK, do you feel like you're ready? I feel like you're ready, your preceptor feels like you're ready. I think if you feel like you're ready, we can go, but do you feel like you like you need more time?" They we're really flexible with that. I said "OK, let me try it on my own!"*

You should feel like the preceptor is there for you, your experience is negotiable, and you are encouraged to ask questions.

A new nurse comments,

*She was a great preceptor from the get-go. I felt like I could go to her and ask any question. It didn't matter. There was never a stupid question, which I think is a big concern for people when they first get on the floor. Maybe that's a stupid question. You don't necessarily feel comfortable asking what you need to ask. But she was really clear and said, "Listen, ask what you need to ask because I don't want you to get on the floor alone and not have asked it, and then you don't know." She was really kind in that way and open. Her technique was really good. I felt confident learning from her.*

A cross section of newly minted nurses suggest that it is essential for preceptors to recognize that all new grads need to do the following:

1. Build up to handle a group of patients and only add more patients when the new grad feels ready.
2. Learn how to speak with a physician. Talking to a physician is intimidating to all new staff. Communicating patient needs in a way that the physician can respond to appropriately takes practice. SBAR is a tool that has assisted new and experienced nurses in getting their patients' problems known and needs met. Don't assume the physician knows about patient changes. If you report a change and feel you are not heard, contact your preceptor or the charge nurse. Recognize that the key to advocating for your patient is to keep the patient at the center, *not your ego:* "Will I feel nervous?" "What if he

yells at me?" or the *physician's ego:* "Will my question mean I am questioning the physician's judgment?" Keep your concern for the patient's safety and well-being at the center of the question.

3. Learn the patient resources and when should you call them in. Usually in orientation the facilities' resources are described, from working with discharge planning to calling in spiritual care. Yet, until you need a resource for a specific patient, the system doesn't click. Keep the list of patient resources handy so when the time comes you will be able to provide support for your patient.

As Anna described,

*The roommate of my patient suffered from dementia. She was rambling and seeking attention and frustrated. I couldn't seem to help her, and I had to go, but I asked her, "Would you like someone to come and pray with you?" It was a long shot, but she said yes, and I figured having someone pay attention to her and bring good energy to the room could do nothing but help and reassure her. We then had the unit clerk put in a call for the chaplain. It was a spiritual intervention, and my preceptor complimented me for thinking of it.*

4. Ask a lot of questions. Staff like when new grads ask questions. Questioning shows that you are interested in being part of the unit and invested in giving appropriate patient care. Don't be discouraged by the few staff members who may be offended by questioning; just ask someone else.

As one new grad said,

*There are certain people I go to if I have a problem. I get to know the people that I trust. There are certain people I know have certain information. They know the labs, they know the disease process really well, and other people know technique really well. And there are some people I don't talk to. It's not that I don't talk to them, but there are some people I don't feel comfortable asking questions just because they are totally disorganized or look stressed out and I don't want to bother them.*

5. Learn how to organize. First-year nurses report,
   • *The thing is, in the beginning you do not know your own style yet, like how to organize, how to get through the shift.*

- *I observed other nurses: how to organize report sheets; I needed to find one that works.*

- *It took me awhile to realize that I am not going to remember everything. I have to write everything down.*

- *No one is going to remember everything. With an eye toward patient safety, all nurses write things down.*

It has been said for 30 years that novice nurses are task oriented. Yet in the *First Year Study,* the senior nursing student and novice nurse report that it is their *preceptors* who are very task oriented.

Sarah's preceptor took a different approach:

*"He was not about concentrating on tasks," Sarah wrote. He'd say, "Let's stop and think what is going on with your patient. He has CHF (congestive heart failure), diuresis. What do you expect to see? Crackles, edema?" (That's all I knew.)*

*"OK. Let's go head to toe, head, neck, heart . . . . If he is having problems breathing, what would you do?" So I'd visualize this happening and I felt prepared when I went in to see my patient.*

Now that's a good preceptor! Supervisors offer support too. You should expect helpful interactions with the supervisor, like these new grads experienced:

*Supervisors who were genuine in their interest and gave you the time to be heard were ideal but not typical. Oh, on paper it would say the supervisor would check-in, but that check-in was interpreted by some supervisors as a wave and "how ya doin'?"; others took the time.*

*My supervisor is really good too. He has been really good at checking in with me to make sure I'm feeling comfortable. He does rounding on all the nurses, once a month. He has them come in for 5 to 10 minutes and asks, "Are you having any issues, any problems, do you need anything?" He also has lunch with us. He's very friendly.*

The charge nurse or the resource nurse should be there for you too:

*There's a charge nurse during the week. She's been a nurse for 25 years, and I go to her all the time. She makes it part of her job to be really supportive to the new grads. I don't know if it is technically part of her job description. She makes it part of her job. She always checks in with us. She makes sure we're doing what we need to do and asks if we have any questions.*

New nurses also bring something to the table. Beckett, Gilbertson, & Greenwood (2007) observed that it is difficult for new nurses to see the value they bring to their practice because they become so preoccupied with their perceived lack of knowledge and technical skills. The authors remind us that: "Despite their feelings of deficit, they are effectively negotiating relational ethics (p. 28)." New graduates learned how to form nurse-patient relationships during their clinical rotations. They report thinking holistically until they got on the floor and were confronted with a list of tasks that was 10 miles long.

All of the nurses make a difference. One new grad told me that the team of nurses that new nurses work with can "make or break" their experiences. He described some of his coworkers as "micromanaging newer nurses" and stated that generally these nurses are the ones he has less respect for regarding their skills. The story of bonding with the nurse would not be complete without recognizing that it is possible to land in a place where there is a lack of connection.

# WHAT IF THERE IS NO CONNECTION?

You have to look out for this problem of not feeling like you belong. As with any profession, there is the underside of nursing behavior where the staff appear to be unwelcoming, intimidating, and sometimes bullying. Brian, a new grad, just returned from a successful job interview. When he went to interview he wanted to work in the intensive care unit (ICU), but after meeting each staff on two different units he said he could feel the difference between the two units. One unit was enthusiastic and welcoming; the other seemed like a closed system that would be difficult to break into. Although he had applied for the ICU, he chose the other unit because he said, "My priority is to look forward to going to work everyday."

Sharon reported,

*Since graduating from the second bachelor's program, I started on a position in the medical surgical unit and realized quickly that the environment was unwelcoming to new grads. Perhaps I should emphasize that the environment*

*was unwelcoming to new grads with voices. I felt that what was more impor-*
*tant than learning how to function as a nurse was being able to take on the*
*high patient load and that was what nursing was all about at that facility.*

*I was still on orientation when I finally gave my notice. I was up to five*
*patients and was about to increase that load to six, not by choice. I had stated*
*on a few occasions that I felt I needed to know more about the patients in*
*order to really care for them, but that went out of the window. So I was run-*
*ning around, not really learning anything and most importantly, not having*
*an opportunity to read the patients' charts, to review histories, any of that.*
*To sum it all up, I finally gave my notice about a month ago, mainly because*
*I felt the environment was unsafe for patients and for new nurses.*

*Next, I applied at a home-care agency and I am currently working as the*
*pediatric home-care nurse. What a difference! I not only enjoy caring for pedi-*
*atric clients, but I now have the opportunity to get to know my clients and*
*read about their histories and medical backgrounds. I can review their 485s*
*(charts) and asked tons of questions. This, I think, is so important in caring*
*for patients. How can you effectively care for patients without looking at the*
*whole person?*

Dee recognizes,

*It has often been said that "nurses eat their young," and there is certainly*
*some truth to this adage. However, the majority of seasoned nurses love to*
*teach and to facilitate growth among junior staff. The new nurse needs to be*
*able to distinguish between these two types and to spend as much time as pos-*
*sible in the company of the second group.*

Both Brian and Sharon experienced how important it is to have a sense
of connection, a welcoming atmosphere, and a friendly staff. They each
described the culture of their unit as critical. The *First Year Study* participants identified culture as an essential element for the new grad to succeed.

# CONCLUSION

As poet David Whyte observed, we feel better when we belong. You want
to start your first job as a nurse where you feel welcomed, attended to, and

recognized. These are reasonable expectations. In nursing, the new nurse is expected to care for his or her own patients soon after being hired. You have as much responsibility as the 20-year nurse next to you, so you must feel supported and connected to your colleagues so you can build your confidence gradually and develop your competence over time. This is your license, your career. Take good care of it so you can give the best care to your patients.

# References

Beckett, A., Gilbertson, S., & Greenwood, S. (2007). Doing the right thing: nursing students, relational practice, and moral agency. *Journal of Nursing Education.* *46*(1), 28–32.

Chandler, G. (1991). Creating an empowered environment. *Nursing Management,* *22*(8),20–23.

Gladwell, M. (2005). *Blink.* NY: Little, Brown & Co.

Nurse Executive Center, The Advisory Board (2006). Transitioning new graduates to hospital practice.

Roche, J., Morsi, D., & Chandler, G. (2009). Testing a work environment–work relationship model to explain expertise in experienced acute care nurses. *Journal of Nursing Administration.* *39*(3), 115–122.

Whyte, D. (1997). *There is no house like a house of belonging (Poem).* Langley, WA: Many Rivers Press.

# [CHAPTER 7]

# Culture

*Culture is like wealth; it makes us more ourselves, it enables us to express ourselves.*

—Philip Gilbert Hamerton

A culture of a country, a town, or a nursing unit is described as a way of being that everyone knows but the rules are unwritten. It's like driving a car. When you first learn to drive you follow all the rules, but then the use of the turn signal, deciphering road signs, and knowing the location of speed traps becomes automatic: You learn the culture of driving. There are unwritten rules for driving, but everybody knows what they are. Likewise, students pick up the culture of a unit fast. They can tell if the nurses are welcoming or if they see students as a burden. I am sure you have had a clinical where the welcoming culture or the "students are a burden" culture, is predominant. It is not hard to tell. But in an interview, where you are primarily concerned about the impression you are making, it may be difficult to focus on the impression the unit is making on you. It is critical, however, for your success in your new job, for you to get a sense of the culture of the unit you will be working on. Recently a senior student, on returning from a very successful interview, reported he knew right away which unit would be friendlier to a new grad and which unit he would not look forward to working on every day. It is possible to get a read on the culture just by visiting the floor, if you know what to look for.

The culture of the unit can be learned by observing how the staff communicate with each other, how the nurse relates to patients, the staff's attitude at change of shift, and the general feel of the unit. The unit culture affects how we feel about our job and how we care for our patients. We know that how we perform in any job is influenced by the environment we work in and by the people we work with. On the units where staff members have good relationships with each other, where timely patient information is provided (not at the moment before admission or discharge), and where there are opportunities to build skills, we feel more comfortable and gain confidence. We feel empowered to function at our best. An environment structured for empowerment has these characteristics:

1. Relationships that work
2. Information that fits
3. Opportunities for growth

Relationships, information, and opportunities are what you want to look for. Did you notice that with your nursing instructors? Your level of competence was affected by the instructor's approach and his or her attitude toward teaching and learning. The instructor you felt you had a good relationship with, who provided the class with organized information and who planned opportunities for you to learn, is the one with whom you felt the best. Then when you went to clinical, the floor's acceptance of students influenced your confidence. On a floor that had the know-how and welcomed the opportunity to teach students, you felt like you could fly! You felt safe enough to try new skills, calm enough to think through what was going on with the patient, and actually thought, "I can do this!" Then, with other instructors or on units where the staff were unwelcoming, you felt intimidated, nervous, deflated, and seriously questioned your ability to be a nurse. Well, the same goes for working. The work environment dramatically affects your functioning. When considering a place to work, look for these qualities:

- *Culture of connection*: respectful relationships, good communication, and staff collaboration.
- *Culture of inquiry*: information is shared, questions are welcome, new ideas are sought, and evidence is used.
- *Culture of quality of life*: refers to the quality of life of the staff. Is the patient load manageable? Are there opportunities for learning? Are the schedules reasonable? Is holiday time negotiable?

Keep this central question in mind: "What will empower you to do your best?" You want to make sure the environment where you choose to work is structured for empowerment.

# CULTURE OF CONNECTION

The previous chapter on bonding emphasized how important a sense of belonging is to new grads. We are social beings. The worst punishment possible is to put prisoners in isolation. It is devastating to be disconnected from others. In any new job we want to have a positive connection to our peers, preceptors, and the health-care team. Let's face it. You have just left one of the closest connections of your life: college. Whether you got together for fun, collaborated over a class conflict, or carpooled to clinical, college afforded the time to nurture friendships. Work is a whole different story. In your new job you will figure out how to develop new friends and confidants, how to develop your communication skills so you can collaborate with other health-care providers, and how to quiet all the other demands in your new role so you can establish a connection with your patients.

To assist new grads in adjusting to the work culture, some hospitals provide opportunities for new nurses from different units to meet with each other. Through purposely designed group meetings where narratives of practice are shared, case studies are analyzed, and personal doubts are voiced, new nurses develop a support network. Other facilities have formally taught preceptors about coaching and mentoring, the importance of encouraging their novice nurses and the necessity of offering positive feedback. The preceptor connection that works well goes beyond teaching/learning and provides opportunities to discuss the disappointment in feeling a lack of competence, the fear that you won't know what symptoms to look for, or the worry that you won't know how to anticipate what will happen next. To support the preceptor connection, socializing is encouraged, downtime is set aside, and food is provided. No matter how well prepared you feel, the whole world looks better through the lens of connection.

A new nurse reports,

*From the beginning, my preceptor always made it a point to include me in the social stuff, which sounds silly, but I think it makes a big difference. The usual way the nurses behave makes new grads feel isolated. New grads don't have any camaraderie and they're new grads, so no one wants to hang out with them. But she made a point. She would say, "Come sit over here and have lunch with us." She kind of integrated me into the floor socially, which is important. She was liked on the floor, which kind of made me well liked by association.*

Now that is a thoughtful preceptor! It just occurred to me that a downside of 12-hour shifts may be that when you finally get out of work you are too exhausted to do anything else together. Going out after an 8-hour, 3 to 11 shift, was what got me through my first job. I remember walking out onto the steps of West House after a particularly grueling shift when someone suggested we all go out for a beer. I was still so new, my first thought was "But what about my homework?" Then I realized I didn't have any! So off we went to Harvard Square for an unofficial staff debriefing and stress reliever. If you work 12-hour shifts, you will have to make room for time to socialize. Both common sense and research evidence support the fact that if you are more comfortable with each other, the work will flow more easily and outcomes will improve. Health care is very concerned about outcomes and preventing errors. Recent research identified stressors that related to the lack of connection:

- Inconsistent support from preceptors, managers, and educators
- Lack of confidence in communicating with physicians
- Fear of caring for patients who are dying
- Lack of support from ancillary personnel (Fink, Casey, Krugman, & Goode, 2008)

This makes sense. In a work environment that is structured to empower the staff, the evidence recognizes the importance of vertical and lateral relationships (Chandler, 1992; Cho, Laschinger, & Wong, 2006; Kanter, 1986). In one of the best jobs I ever had, we did excellent work and had a lot of fun (that is possible!). The nurses, social workers, and physicians met in daily rounds where we worked intently to develop treatment plans for very complex patients. Through our regular collaboration we developed great working relationships that filtered down to excellent patient care. Although we worked on a unit with very challenging patients, I believe the patients knew we had a smooth running team with consistent communication about approaches to treatment that led to better outcomes. Support from supervisors above, from peers laterally, and from assistive staff below provides a basis for increasing your competence and confidence. The culture of the unit you work on will help you not only survive but thrive in nursing. Or, the culture can work against you.

Here is how Nancy had both experiences in one shift:

*Originally I started out my day with my usual preceptor, but she had to leave the shift so another nurse was assigned to my patients and me. I thought she was a bit aloof and rude to me. I found her completely unnerving and very judgmental. As a result, I found myself making stupid mistakes such as forgetting supplies, charting, and answers to questions I knew. At lunch I learned that she was a local community college instructor on Fridays, so all of her intrusive comments from the morning made more sense. After lunch, another nurse, whom I found was much better to work with, took over my patients. Although she had floated all over the hospital that day and was worn out, she still found enough energy to be kind and teach me. We made a good team for the rest of the day. It was good for me to experience this week's confusion and unexpected changes along with the rudeness of the college instructor. I learned how just one person can radically alter your experience depending on their style and approach.*

Interdisciplinary teamwork, well documented as the ideal for efficient functioning, patient safety, and quality patient outcomes, is seen as essential but not necessarily present on every unit. The truth is that good nursing care is very difficult without collaborative teamwork. The problems patients present are much too complex for one nurse or one discipline to manage alone. The reason a patient comes into the hospital is to be assessed, diagnosed, and managed by a team of care providers. Think about it: People with health problems acute enough to be admitted to the hospital are going to present with complex issues. Then isolate them from their family and friends, include a lot of poking and prodding, order tests and blood draws, offer a handful of medication, and then move them to a strange and uncomfortable setting where they are no longer in control of even going to the bathroom, and this is where the nurse comes in. Your patients are already well out of their comfort zone when you walk in the room. That's where the nurse has to take the lead in creating a positive environment for patients. Managing the individual patient and contributing the health-care team is a big role for a new nurse to assume.

A recent grad had these practical recommendations on contributing to a positive culture:

*I credit my positive feelings to the positive team culture that I feel is present on the unit, which I try to contribute to. Here are some recommendations:*

- *Try to imagine every patient is a family member.*
- *Always do your own assessment—don't prejudge a patient based on report information.*
- *It's not just about your patients, it's about the whole team.*
- *You are not going to be the most experienced nurse right away—you have to go through the process, the crap, the experiences to get there.*

- *Recognize that skills take practice. I learned that doing the skills "over and over again" is what I need to build them. I realize that this takes time, but I feel positive that I will continue to gain the skills I cannot do independently.*
- *You owe it to your patients to develop a positive attitude. Think, "I am as important as any member of the team, I am a nurse."*
- *Have a little faith and be proud of your achievements.*

In other words, take care of yourself and attend to your attitude. One way to do this is to take a moment to take a deep breath before you enter a patient's room. There is so much going on in our heads that sometimes the patient gets lost. We are thinking about the disease process, the symptoms, the patient's history, the presenting problem, and anticipating the next step. We are considering the person's physiological, psychological, cognitive, spiritual, and familial response. We are dealing with the patient's attitude, energy level, learning capacity, economic limitations, and outlook on life. When we are just starting, we tend to be more focused on the tasks that have to be completed: vital signs, meds, and dressing changes, rather than the whole patient. In the beginning we can get tunnel vision.

A nurse out of school for 6 months writes,

*One of the things I remember most about Luke is his parents. Taking care of Luke was one of the first times when I had started to see beyond the patient— the immediate task at hand—to the family surrounding the patient. When I first started nursing, my vision was so tunneled; I could barely see the patient I was performing procedures on. I used to joke with my preceptor that there could be a fire at the next bedside, and I probably wouldn't even notice it because I was so completely focused on that lung I was listening to.*

*I think one of my biggest regrets about caring for Luke is the nagging feeling that I wasn't there enough for the family. Besides not knowing what to say, I was too busy to spend much time with them. I answered their questions and kept them updated on the plan of care, but I don't think I was there for them emotionally. I remember at change of shift watching and listening to the more experienced day nurse talking to the parents, and it suddenly struck me that they needed me too. Their need was clear to me again during the code. I watched my experienced colleagues pushing drugs and doing compressions while comforting the family at the same time. I realized I was missing a vital component of nursing. There is an art and science to nursing—one of the reasons that drew me to nursing—and I had been focusing all my energies on*

*the science side. I knew that to be a truly competent nurse, I would also need
to start focusing on the art of nursing. When art and science are blended
together perfectly, you can be there for both the patients and their families.*

Although we are assigned to a group of patients, we cannot manage
care alone. We are dealing with too much to think of everything. We need
input and assistance from our peers and the other members of the health-
care team. The social worker, chaplain, pharmacist, and wound specialist
are resources to be tapped. The nurse is at the hub of this expansive wheel,
at the hub, with the patient.

Communication is the first step to interdisciplinary collaboration. To
collaborate with the physician, good nurse/doctor communication is
required. Communicating with physicians takes practice, and it is one of
the skills nurses have agreed that they do not get enough practice with in
school. Look for opportunities to be the nurse who contacts the physician.
Taking initiative begins with a supportive preceptor and other staff nurses
that role-model effective professional interactions. Communication tools,
such as SBAR (Situation, Background, Assessment, Recommendation) can
assist nurses in organizing data, reflecting on their thoughts, and developing their suggestions so they can paint a complete picture when communicating with the physician. Good communication occurs one person at a time.

Nancy had this experience recently:

*What I found interesting about this patient was the collaboration that
occurred between the patient's doctor, my preceptor, and me. We were deeply
concerned for the patient and his decline. He is married and a father of two
children. They were often in to visit. The doctor did an exemplary job of communicating with the wife and updating her on her husband's care via tele-
phone and in person. The doctor was approachable and open to suggestions.
Emotionally it was important for us to not let this condition get out of control.
I found myself exhibiting boldness and independence from my preceptor by
taking the opportunity to talk with the doctor about my concerns. I questioned
administering a dose of Toradol originally ordered by the attending covering
for the doc. The doc withheld it because the patient had an elevated creatinine
level. This experience brought the doctor and me closer. These past 2 weeks he
has been much more receptive to engaging in conversations with me regarding
patients. This had not been the case before this experience. This patient
brought us into a situation where conversation was incredibly important, and
it helped break down student, doctor, and nurse barriers. We are all people, and
we should do what we can for each other.*

Sounds like solid advice. Looks to me like the improvement in communication occurred through the nurse knowing the details of the situation and speaking up while recognizing the importance of everyone's role on the team.

Collaborating with the nursing assistant is another essential dynamic that contributes to the success of the nursing role and patient care. You all know the five rights of delegation:

1. The right task
2. Under the right circumstances
3. To the right person
4. With the right directions and communication
5. Under the right supervision and evaluation

The American Nurses Association (ANA) and the National Council of State Boards of Nursing (NCSBN) (2005) wrote a comprehensive paper on delegation that describes the process, necessity, and legal implications (http://www.ncsbn.org.). Delegation begins with the ability to be assertive. Whether communicating with a physician, a certified nursing assistant (CNA), or a nursing peer, assertiveness techniques can be useful tools.

Sarah had a situation in the beginning where she wished she was more assertive and had talked to her preceptor:

*A CNA told me I had no right to delegate to her. This was very upsetting. I did not know how to handle it. Now I wish I had had more opportunity to talk about conflict management and delegation in school.*

Conflict management and assertiveness go together. Both take practice. Being assertive to advocate for your patient and to stand up for yourself is so central to success in professional practice. Here is a quick lesson.

Assertiveness is a learned behavior. With practice we can all improve our assertive communication. For some it looks like assertiveness comes naturally, but that is because they learned it early. As with any new learning experience, you have to practice. With assertiveness you can practice by using scripts. This is nothing new. In any relationship where we anticipate a challenging verbal exchange, we naturally go over a script in our head, like when we are going to confront our boyfriend or girlfriend about an important issue or how we are going bring up a touchy topic with our parents. We usually obsess about the conversation by rehearsing it over and over in our head. So scripting out a conversation in advance is nothing new. These are the three assertiveness steps:

1. "I understand"
2. "I need"
3. "Let's talk"

For example, you want to ask to change a shift:

> "*I* understand *the evening shift needs to be covered, but I* need *to attend my sister's wedding rehearsal dinner. Can we* talk *about the best way to fill my position?*"

Let the person know you get what the needs are but you have needs too, and then you invite conversation. A friend has been late picking you up for work:

> "*I UNDERSTAND we have to get up early and it takes a lot of planning to get out of the house when you have young children. However, this is a new job for me and I am just learning, so in order to be prepared to take care of my patients, I NEED to be there 15 minutes early. CAN WE TALK about how to make this happen?*"

Or talking to a CNA who has worked at the facility much longer than you:

> "*I UNDERSTAND that you know the unit routine much better than I do which is great. However, I NEED to know the vital signs by 8 o'clock so I can anticipate what meds to prepare. LET'S TALK about how we can work this out.*"

Practice the three steps in your own life: "I understand," "I need," "let's talk," before you use assertiveness at work, or getting your roommate to do the dishes. You'll be surprised at the positive response you get or at least a beginning conversation.

> "*I UNDERSTAND you are very busy and you are always on the run, but I NEED to have the kitchen a bit neater so I feel like eating here too. It's not that appetizing with the sink full of dirty dishes. CAN WE TALK about how to share the dish responsibility?*"

A component of assertiveness to keep in mind is using "I" and not "you." When you start using "you" like "*You* weren't on time," or "*You* made me late," the person gets defensive. Try to stay with "I" messages.

Communication, or rather poor communication, is the number-one threat to patient safety. Being good at communicating takes daily practice, and then there will still be times when you will walk away wishing you said something differently. Recently Rachael asked the staff why there was such poor communication between nurses and nurses, nurses and doctors, and nurses and patients. This is what she heard:

1. The newer nurses have a lack of confidence that held them back from saying anything they thought would cause a problem for fear they would be labeled troublemakers or ostracized.
2. The nurses who had been there longer agreed there was a problem but now they accept "that is just how it is," and it is easier to function if you make less waves.
3. Many felt if they spoke up it would either add too much stress or they would be labeled.

This is frightening for all concerned. We cannot afford the potential errors silence could incur or the waste of time work-arounds take when system change is necessary Developing your voice is essential to your success. Today we have so much instant communication, I find I need to remind myself to stop all I am doing and just listen. I have to be mindful of the person and the situation. We have been trained to be distracted, to multitask. It takes practice to pay attention, listen to others, and listen to ourselves. Jenni is paying attention to her patient, and the cues she gets from herself in response to the patient to know what to do next:

*Mrs. W was a familiar face to me at the hospice home since I had been assigned to care for her the 2 previous weeks. Our first meeting had left me emotionally and physically drained due to the effort on the part of myself, the head nurse, and Mrs. W's daughter to keep her from inadvertently hurting herself as she writhed in pain from end-stage pancreatic and bone cancer. In her mid-80s, I instantly observed the wasting away of her body that was apparent in her sunken eyes, prominent cheekbones, and protruding hip bones that were evident through her faded Johnny and the excess skin that collected at her elbows. In response to the pain, Mrs. W thrashed aimlessly and fitfully as I strategically placed pillows against the bed rails and secured her Johnny in such a way that prevented her from becoming entangled or possibly choking herself. I was attentive to Mrs. W's actions in response to the morphine pump dose being adjusted by her nurse. I knew that the decreased liver function in elder adults offers a delicate balance between too little and too much pain medication. For someone who appeared so frail and weak, the forceful response of her body alternating between rigidity and frailty was astounding. She couldn't speak coherently and yet she managed to cry out in terse phrases with a writhing voice "Mother! . . . Mother Mary!" with painful bouts of "Why have you forsaken . . .?" Then she said one nearly inaudible word: "Pray."*

*I made the association between several pieces of information such as the report of her fall out of bed, her daughter mentioning her mother's sudden devotion to the church, my experience with Mrs. W crying out "Mother Mary," and the presence of her rosary on the bedside table. I realized that she was trying to get out of bed in order to assume a position of prayer. Knowing this was not safe, I gently gained her attention by speaking her name. I held her hand, and looking at her distraught face I soothingly spoke to her. "You don't have to get out of bed to pray." Mrs. W stopped moving and focused her attention on me, her confused eyes searching my face. "No?" she replied. "No," I said. "God can hear you pray while you're lying down."*

*She remained still and I observed her actions. It was as if she had never considered this option as she slowly leaned back against the pillows. I also told her that we needed to keep her covered because it was one of those cool fall mornings. She lifted her eyes to mine and I sensed she understood. If it were possible, I would swear that I saw her flash back to another time in her life where she remembered that kind of morning on her family's orchard farm. I pulled the covers up over her and adjusted her pillows as I described how it was still apple-picking season and how the colors were changing, and the air was getting cooler. Even though Mrs. W's failing sight did not allow her to see all the things I saw coming into the hospice home that morning, I at least could describe them to her. And that brought her peace. I asked her if she wanted her rosary. She nodded affirmatively, and I had my fellow student obtain it while she turned on some soothing music. Mrs. W didn't have the coordination to maintain a grasp on her rosary beads, so I held them in her hand while she closed her eyes. I observed her mouth moving without sound and considered her to be in prayer. She became calm, and after a few minutes, she was in a peaceful slumber.*

Jenni was paying attention, mindful of her patient and mindful of her own reactions. It takes practice to clear your head of the constant self-talk on what you should have done or what you still have to do. Our mind is like a bus. We carry a lot of passengers up there demanding our time and attention, voices from our parents, "Make sure you are on time"; voices from the present, "Remember your paper is due on Friday"; and voices from the future, "When should I go back to grad school?" The good news is you are old enough to drive that bus and be in charge. You can tell who to get off. That takes practice too. It takes 5 to 10 minutes of quiet to begin. I know you don't have time. But if you are not going to listen to you, who will? Besides, it is interesting to observe what voices come up. Have you tried to meditate? Just sit still for 5 minutes and pay attention to your breath. Wait until you see how distracted you are with other thoughts. It takes practice to still those voices.

One of my friends says she cannot meditate because too many thoughts come up. Well, that's the point: to become aware of all those voices in your head so you can learn how to quiet them when you need to pay attention and be present. Presence is one of the most valuable approaches a nurse can offer to her patient. Patients have reported that being present is healing. We know this already from our own experience. Take a moment to recall the last time you were talking to a good friend who was really present and listening attentively. Who was your friend? What were you talking about? What did that experience feel like? It felt like your friend really wanted to understand what was going on and empathized with your situation, right? Being listened to attentively is a rewarding experience. That's what you can do for patients. Nurses can have a healing presence. You probably have already noticed the power of presence when you were in nursing school taking care of your patients. Now you just have to practice being present with yourself first, so you can bring this gift to others, just as Jenni did.

In addition to learning how to actively listen, the new nurse is expected to ask a lot of questions. You want to question things you are not sure of, question things you do not understand, question things you don't think are quite right. That is how you learn. The only stupid question is the one not asked. You want to work in a place where everyone questions, where everyone thinks critically, where there is a culture of inquiry.

# CULTURE OF INQUIRY

"I don't have a shift where I don't ask another nurse a question or don't ask someone for help." This quote is not from a new nurse but from one of our top clinical instructors who is an Emergency Department expert. Questioning is key to critical thinking, and safe practice. Questioning is the basis for new learning. We can find answers on our own by reviewing policies and procedures or searching the evidence or simply asking a colleague.

Sarah, a new nurse, observed,

*Even the experienced nurses learn new things all the time and ask for help. The nurses on my floor have told me time and again that they will be there to support me as a new nurse.*

A culture of inquiry is required for your learning, the staff's development (they too learn from every question you ask), and for your patient's health. The culture of the unit can encourage your growth or stifle your progress. You'll know from the start whether you feel included, which tells you a lot about how your questions will be received. When you are on an interview, assess the culture by considering:

1. Are your questions welcome?
2. Are your questions answered?
3. Do the floor nurses use evidence to support their practice?
4. Is the evidence you present welcomed?
5. Ask yourself if the dominant attitude is open and interested in what you bring to the table or is it "our way or the highway?"

Today's graduate comes from an educational program whose mission is to develop critical thinkers. New nurses are trained to reflect on their practice and ask questions about what they do not know, what seems unusual, and what they have not encountered before. A nurse 6 months out reported,

*Even today I still ask questions, I never feel shy asking the questions. Everybody does, everybody asks questions, because there will always be something you don't know. Everyone is receptive to questions. That's on the up side.*

*As I am coming up on 6 months, I find myself asking fewer questions, feeling more confident.*

Sometimes, questions are experienced as criticizing a nurse's practice rather than a way of learning how the nurse is thinking by asking the nurse to think out loud. You may have to make your critical thinking style known to the nurse you are questioning. Second-year bachelor's students tend to question everything because before nursing they excelled in other responsible positions, so they recognize the amount of responsibility on a nurse's shoulders. One senior, in her internship, asked a lot of questions to her preceptor that came off as the preceptor feeling like the student was questioning her practice. I had the student intern explain to the preceptor that questioning is how she learns. Her questions are not questioning the preceptor's practice but rather trying to understand how actual practice fits with what she had been taught in school. In most cases the intern was asking the preceptor to think out loud so she could see how the preceptor arrived at decisions. Nurses pick up new information by asking questions.

*Anytime I am unsure about something or haven't seen something done yet, I just go to whoever is around and there's a wealth of seasoned nurses. I can ask anyone; they talk me through it. People are happy to do it. Also, there is a really good clinical nurse specialist. Unfortunately, I work a lot of weekends so I don't always get that resource available all the time. If I work during the week, I go to her.*

The majority of staff nurses feel more comfortable if you are asking questions. They know you are new and don't know much yet so they expect you to speak up. Questioning physicians brings a whole other level of ability:

*The thing that I felt skittish about was paging the doctors because I didn't want to look like an idiot. They are also very good; no one made me feel like an idiot.*

*I just had that fear that I don't want to ask stupid questions, but guess what? I do ask stupid questions. It's just a part of being new and that is OK.*

Inquiring through questioning will develop your knowledge and skills. Finding evidence through academic Web sites and valid published research to answer your questions will increase your competence and lead to establishing a practice based on evidence, a necessity and professional expectation in our informational society.

An evidenced-based practice is required for all health-care providers. Often new grads are more adept at locating evidence than the more experienced nurses. All facilities are aware of the necessity of basing practice on evidence. This is a skill you bring to your new position. You know how to locate evidence from the most recent literature to support your opinions and the latest research, an ability that is critical to provide the most effective patient care.

Anna choose a project that would benefit the unit:

*I noticed how hard it was with three patients to keep track of I/Os (intakes and outtakes). I found two articles in a quick search that I wanted to further consider, one by McConnell (2002) talks about do's and dont's in a broad task-like way, and another by Wise, Emrsch, Racioppi, Crosier, & Thompson (2000) that concludes that I and O is unreliable even when done well.*

The next vignette describes the process used by Ann to base her practice on valid evidence:

*Due to the low amniotic fluid index (AFI), the patient had an order for continuous fetal monitoring until her C-section the next morning. I didn't know my AFI values, so I asked the nurse I was working with that shift. She didn't know them either, but I was a little concerned that instead of going to a reference text or a journal article, she Googled it and picked the first article, which wasn't from an academic source. I was also concerned about how she interpreted the information from the article, so I decided I should find another source for a better idea as to how serious this patient's level might be. From an academic source I learned that even at AFI levels of 5 to 10 cm, there is a significantly increased association with adverse perinatal outcome, so my patient's level of 4.2 cm, indeed, needed to be taken seriously.*

You know how to search Web sites that are based on valid research, including in-house resources. In this case Anna's quest for better patient tools was met by searching the in-house site:

*The way we were assessing the demented patient's pain was unsatisfactory to me. Therefore, I asked my preceptor if there were other pain scales we could use for nonverbal or cognitively impaired patients. She didn't know where to point me, so I used the hospital's information system and studied a brief PowerPoint presentation about the pain scales available. It was great! I showed my preceptor how there are a multitude of scales on the Web site, including Wong-Baker, Infant and Pedi, and the PAINAD and the scale for nonverbal, cognitively impaired adults. This scale used criteria like facial expressions, movement, moaning, etc., to determine a pain scale number. This helped me advocate for stronger pain medication for my patient. Score 1 for patient and 1 for new nurse!*

Now, not that we want to keep score, but you do bring important skills to your new job. Here's another example of what the next generation adds to the picture:

*I had a great example of how students can teach RNs on the floor. We were talking about certain blood pressure medications and I was asking about ethnic considerations for certain drugs. My nurse was unaware that certain genetic factors made people process drugs in different ways. I explained to her about the example of asparagus and the enzyme that makes one's urine smell unusual after eating it. She, not having that enzyme, didn't know about this and was amazed to learn such a concrete example of how genetics really do affect how people process drugs and the clinical implications thereof.*

Way to go, Anna! You are smart too. It is just that being new makes you feel dumb. But if you find a work culture that facilitates connections and encourages inquiry, you will find your north star and find a place where you fit. Life is not just about work, though. To meet all of these new expectations you have to have a work/life balance.

# A CULTURE OF QUALITY OF LIFE: YOURS!

Because quality of life and work/life balance came up as stressors in two recent surveys of new nurses, we should talk about it (Fink et al., 2008; Halfer & Graf, 2006). We know nursing care is provided for patients 24/7, 365 days a year. That is why patients go to the hospital, so they can be monitored by nurses around the clock. That was also part of the attraction to nursing: always on the go, standing by, ready for the next patient. That's thrilling on TV, but what about if this expectation of always being at attention, accepting, and caring is your life?

Fink et al. (2008) reported two groups of stressors: the first 6 months and from 6 to 12 months.

The first 6 months:

1. Taking the National Council Licensure Examination for Registered Nurses (NCLEXRN) and waiting to hear
2. Moving away from home
3. Adjusting to a new work environment

The next 6 to 12 months:

1. Family responsibilities
2. Becoming married or pregnant
3. Finding a new apartment or house
4. Attending graduate school

OK, now that we know what the stressors are, let's do something about them. Being aware of work requirements is key to managing your life and having some quality, hopefully a lot of quality! Your work schedule, holiday time, and work/life balance impact your life.

## Schedules

Every nursing unit has a schedule that may or may not rotate between shifts and probably has seniority preferences. You need to find out what the shift rotation is. The new person is most likely to be at the bottom of the seniority totem pole. So what exactly will that mean for your life? That is the question you need to ask your interviewer and yourself. Is it a rule that new staff work nights until someone retires? Are you expected to rotate between days and nights? Evenings and nights? How often?

Several *First Year Study* participants reported that on hire, nights was their only option. Tammi told us that initially she couldn't imagine how she would adjust her sleep patterns, her relationship, or her exercise routine. Several nurses reported, however, that after orienting on days and witnessing the nonstop chaos, they were relieved to be on the night shift where they could actually think, plan, then respond, and reflect.

Amanda reported,

*I like nights. I get to plan what I am going to do, I look things up, I have time to think and plan. There is time to look up policies, meds, and evidence. I learned how to maximize my organization through prioritizing and I never feel on my own. We help each other out. It is too hectic on days.*

Tammi confessed,

*I had never even stayed up all night. I was in a new marriage and couldn't imagine what 10-hour nights would be like. But, after 6 months, they work for me. The night staff are super supportive, and they love to teach. I do get to look things up. I have figured out how to get to my exercise class, have a sleep schedule, and use my days off to recover. It is okay for now. I will have the opportunity to change in a couple of months, but I think I'll stay put. I really like the people I work with.*

Any new schedule can wreak havoc with your biorhythms and your lifestyle. Getting up at 5:30 a.m. to get to the day shift can be exhausting for many, or getting out at 11:30 p.m. can limit your time with family and friends.

Claudia told me,

*The requirement to work evenings is what led to me moving to a new position. I had been married for 25 years and missed evenings with my husband and friends.*

What work schedule would fit in with your lifestyle, or how can you adjust your life to fit work? When you are asked about your preferences, you want to be prepared to answer. Before you sign on, you will want to know the time you will work and the time you will have off.

# Holidays

We have been trained since birth to anticipate holidays. From kindergarten on, our school schedule reinforced vacation times around holidays. Now being a nurse, all those rituals we have assumed are out the window. We could be scheduled for Thanksgiving Day and Christmas Eve, or July Fourth and New Year's Day. Some nurses take the holiday expectation in stride, but others experience increased stress. Find out what the holiday policy is. Talk to other nurses about how to adjust, secrets to managing family expectations, and hints on how to cope with work requirements. Talk to your family about job expectations and how to work together to keep up traditions or make some adjustments.

# Work/Life Balance

You need it! Deepak Chopra (1990) said: Balance is what it is all about. Being out of balance leads to stress and illness. Rest, exercise, nutrition, and good relationships need to be balanced with work.

You figured how to juggle all those school requirements, so you know you can do it. This is a great conversation to have with other new grads or nurses who have been out a year or two. How do you keep up? A friend of mine studied nurses who were considered the experts by their colleagues. These experts were nominated by their peers. When Sue flew out to meet with the expert staff nurses, she found their schedules hard to pin down. Either they were very busy on the job with no time for an interview or on their days off they were gone. I mean, they were nowhere to be found. When the expert nurses left work, they left town for the beach or the mountains. Later, in analyzing the data, Sue realized getting far away from work contributed to being able to be an expert while at work. When the expert nurses were at work they were intensely, fully involved, completely present with their patients and responsive to their peers. When they were off they were off recovering, replenishing, nurturing their bodies, minds, and spirits. There is a lesson in here for all of us. Learn from your mentor, preceptor, and peers how to create your own work/life balance so you can maintain a positive attitude. Sometimes, when things don't go right, a negative culture can develop.

# THE NEGATIVE CULTURE

From the hundreds of nursing students I have taught, I have consistently heard that the desire to be a nurse came from the wish to care for others, to assist the most vulnerable, and to focus on the whole person. I have never met a nurse wannabe who said he or she wanted to enter the profession to be unsupportive, to be unhelpful, or to be intimidating. Yet there are nurses who have been described in these pejorative terms. What happened between the optimism of school and the pessimism in the workplace? What happens in the work environment that affects the attitudes and behaviors of the nurse who started out with such good intentions?

Unfortunately, we do not have all the answers. Some suggest the powerlessness that a nurse experiences in the health-care hierarchy erodes individual confidence and professional attitude over time. Others recognize that the low value placed on nursing work and the lack of public recognition of the enormous contribution the nurse makes to health care leads to devaluing the self and eventually devaluing others. Regardless of the rationale for negative behavior, however, there is consensus that bullying, horizontal violence, or intimidation is prevalent in the work environment.

We know that nurse-to-nurse behaviors that feel like psychological bullying creates a negative culture. It can happen with a look, a word, or simply silence. The result of bullying can create a sense of humiliation, a lack of respect, and the feeling of exclusion from the rest of the staff. This psychological harassment can make new nurses feel powerless, which can lead to a lack of self-confidence. Sometimes the dominant group's behavior includes withholding of opportunities, being exclusive, or not sharing information. This type of behavior is often subtle, experienced as being ignored or being left out. Other times intimidation is more direct, with unkind words spoken or being set up to look inept in front of peers and patients. This lack of collegiality leaves the new nurse particularly vulnerable to job stress. Here's the bottom line: This dangerous, negative behavior between nurses can threaten patient safety.

It is important to recognize this is not new behavior. It is an unfortunate part of nursing's legacy, and it is certainly not your fault. The good news is that intimidation is being openly talked about, and there is a growing body of research describing the experience and the negative results, such as increased stress, increased attrition rates, and ultimately a decrease in quality patient care. Today, individual institutions and national organizations are developing policies to address this behavior. The Joint Commission on Accreditation of Healthcare Organizations, the national accrediting agency, requires hospitals to develop a code of conduct and procedures for dealing with ineffective communication.

There are seemingly inconsequential acts that leave an impression on the new nurse. Pay attention to your response so you know it is not in your head but a normal response to an uncomfortable situation.

Melissa conmented,

*My preceptor didn't know I was coming. She knew she was getting an orienteer but did not know when or who I was. There wasn't a big welcome.*

Doris recognized,

*It has often been said that "nurses eat their young" and there is certainly some truth to this adage, and some nurses who fit this cannibalistic model. However, there are also many seasoned nurses who love to teach and to facilitate growth among junior staff. The new nurse needs to be able to distinguish between these two types and to spend as much time as possible in the company of the second group.*

Courtney's experience with her new job did not work out as planned:

*Within a month into my new job at a world renowned teaching hospital I definitely have a story to tell about adjusting to the new role of RN. I think it is important for new nurses to learn that after all the hard work and all the effort they put in to graduate and pass the boards, that they may end up not even liking their first job! For me I am on a cardiac floor and I find that adjusting to RN is the hardest thing I have ever had to do in my life. I no longer have a road map given to me by my instructor telling me what to do and a name tag identifying me as property of the school. Instead I am just the "newbie" as the other nurses on my floor put it, and I am an outsider looking in. The floor I work on isn't anything I expected it to be. Instead of a supportive staff that asks how I am doing and a friendly face to smile back at me as I am rushing to get paperwork done, I get clique-type young women who look at me as if I have taken care of and killed their mother with a medication error.*

*For the first time in my life, I am having a very difficult time befriending my peers. On my floor it seems as if the priority is not caring for patients but gossiping. It is the patients that are getting me through the day and giving me the strength to go into work each day, and if it wasn't for them I do not know what I would do. It is sad that I look at each day with the mantra of "11 more months" and then I can leave. This transition is the transition that not enough nurses talk about but I am sure many feel.*

Peter's story takes the cake and is one we should all learn from:

*I am writing to let you know about my experience as a new nurse in my first year of practice. The nurse I was trained to be is a professional worker, with a highly developed ability to operate among professional workers, including other nurses, physicians, and other specialties, and I was trained to interact in a professional manner with clients. We are trained to act in a moral fashion, and to treat people in the way we would want to be treated. That is not quite how things turned out.*

*The first indication I had that something was wrong was when, in anticipation of finding a job during a nursing shortage, things were not as I expected. Not a single hospital that I applied to returned my phone calls or even acknowledged that I had applied. My attempts to shake loose a response from any of these hospitals were met by a complete lack of reaction. Although jobs were listed, it was as if these places did not need nurses. In one case I brought a printed copy of my resume in person to a hospital that had at least half a dozen open positions listed. The only person working in the personnel department was a receptionist who would not even take my resume. Rather she sent me back out the door and told me my chances would be better if I applied online.*

*Eventually I found a way to bypass the so-called recruiting department, made contact with a department manager at a hospital I had trained at, discussed a position with her, and received a verbal promise of a job. She said I would have to file an application with human resources and she would take care of the rest. After filing my resume and filling out a job application again, I waited to hear and heard nothing. After waiting and calling and calling again I have to admit, never in my 30 years of professional experience had I been treated so poorly. The only reason I persisted in my attempts to gain employment was because I still at that time held on to the idea that there is a nursing shortage and new, well-educated nurses were needed.*

*Once I was in the hospital I underwent a 14-week orientation for my position in critical care. The 8 weeks were intensive classes where I did quite well. The next 6 weeks I worked under a preceptor, after which I was expected to function in the role of an emergency room nurse. The position I held in the ER was a temporary position, which was promised to become permanent. However, at the end of orientation there was no position unless I took a different shift. Instead of doing that, I sought a position elsewhere in the hospital. So at the end of 14 extremely intense weeks of orientation, I began a second orientation in a completely different department. Unfortunately, I chose what is considered to be the busiest floor in the hospital, which ultimately led me to what I hope are my final days as a hospital nurse.*

*Again, I faced an intense 6 weeks of orientation under the guidance of various seemingly random nurses. I was bumped between four nurses during the orientation. After my orientation I did practice as a nurse finally for 6 more weeks. I watched most of the nurses get frazzled, and I heard them all complain of the ridiculous patient load. What became clear to me very quickly is this is every man or woman for him-herself. I measured my requests for help and knew which nurses could tolerate big questions and which ones could only take small ones. If I asked certain nurses big questions, involving helping me set up treatments, they would go to my boss afterward and I would receive a visit from my boss at 3:15 asking me to meet with her. The meetings were always the same. A laundry list of my flaws was reviewed. I knew which nurses would tattle on me to the boss and which ones would not. Never once did I receive any positive feedback in the 8 months of my employment at the hospital. I relied solely on my own internal compass to know I was progressing at a rapid rate. My only goal was to survive the workday that faced me. To my satisfaction I did survive many without incident, but my final day was a perfect storm of acute patients, discharge paperwork, unsupportive nurse colleagues, and accidental oversights on my part. I left the floor not knowing how I could face another day. My boss called and left me a message at home, confirming that I was at a difficult juncture. I knew my boss had once again formed a judgment without discussing matters with me. I knew I would be returning under scrutiny. I knew it was over, regardless of what my boss said to me. When we did speak, I asked her if she could help me with my shortcomings. She simply said no. It was at this point I spoke to the union steward, who said my mistakes were not final events and I should fight it, but my own ethics dictated that I was done.*

Peter left to pursue a position as a community health nurse and has been quite successful.

# CONCLUSION

Getting a sense of the culture of your new job is key to your survival and success. Pay attention to how staff members talk to each other, whether your questions are welcomed, and what your schedule will be because these are all important indicators of the unit culture. To give the best patient care you will need to be in an environment that provides relationships that work well, gives you the information you'll need to do a good job, and offers opportunities for learning and future professional development. This is a lot to manage on an interview but so important for your success. Recall the quote at the beginning of the chapter: "Culture is like wealth; it makes us more ourselves, it enables us to express ourselves." That is the kind of job that you want, a place that values you being yourself. Your unit wants you to be successful and you want to be the best nurse possible, so make sure there is a good fit between your expectations and their culture.

## References

Chandler, G. (1992). The source and process of empowerment. *Nursing Administration Quarterly, 16*(3), 1–4.

Cho, J., Laschinger, H., & Wong, C. (2006). Workplace empowerment, work engagement and organizational commitment of new graduate nurses. *Nursing Leadership, 19*(3), 43–60.

Chopra, D. (1990). *Quantum healing*. New York: Bantam Books.

Fink, R., Casey, K., Krugman, M., & Goode, C. (2008). The graduate nurse experience. *Journal of Nursing Administration, 38*(7/8), 341–348.

Halfer, D., & Graf, E. (2006). New graduates perception of the work experience, *Nursing Economics, 24*(3), 150–155.

Kanter, R. M. (1986). *Men and women of the corporation*. New York: Basic Books.

McConnell, E. A. (2002). Measuring fluid intake and output. *Nursing, 32*(2), 2.

National Council of State Boards of Nursing. (2005). Working with others: A position paper. Chicago.

Wise, L. C., Emrsch, J. Racioppi, H., Crosier, J., & Thompson, C. (2000). Evaluating the reliability and utility of cumulative intake and output. *Journal of Nursing Care Quality, 14*(3), 37-42.

# [CHAPTER 8]

# The Journey

*"Bird by bird, buddy. Just take it bird by bird."*

—Anne Lamott

In Anne Lamott's book *Bird by Bird* (1994), she tells the story of her 10-year-old brother trying to write a report on birds the night before it was due. He had 3 months to write the report. Delaying writing a paper already sounds familiar, right? So her brother was at the kitchen table surrounded by notebooks, pencils, and unopened books on birds. He was near tears "immobilized by the hugeness of the task ahead. Then my father sat down beside him, put his arm around his shoulder and said, bird by bird buddy, take it bird by bird" (p. 19). That is exactly what we are going to do here. We are going to take this journey into nursing one step at time, bird by bird.

The journey to your first nursing position started when you decided on what nursing program to attend. A 2-year associate's degree (AD) program, a 4-year baccalaureate degree (BS) program, or an accelerated second bachelor's program prepare students differently. Yet, all programs must meet the standards for national accreditation and must adequately prepare their students to pass the nursing licensing (NCLEX) exam. Once you have passed the exam, your journey into nursing winds through the job search and walks you through an orientation that will have you out on your own in 3 to 6 months! How exciting (and scary) is that? Some new grads tell me by the end of the 2-month orientation, if they are on a supportive floor where all the nurses answer their questions and act as preceptors, they feel ready to be on their own. Other new nurses said by 6 months they learned how much they did *not* know and needed more support. This is not uncommon. That is why some facilities have designed amazing year-long residency programs that start with a preceptor in orientation, have regular skills classes, require new grads to attend support groups, and assign a mentor to each new nurse after the first 6 months. Residency programs are designed to provide the support a new nurse needs to succeed. If the facility you are looking at does not have an official residency program, read on and learn what is involved in a program so you can look for and request these supports in your new job.

In this chapter we look at what the journey has been like for first-year nurses so you will be prepared to not only survive but thrive in your first year. By being knowledgeable about the opportunities that different facilities have to offer, you will be better prepared to find the place that fits your needs. Plus, in the interview you will be able to inquire about what is in store for your orientation and what support is offered following the first few weeks. Prior to the interview, you will have already considered what type of support you personally will need because you have already reflected back on other transitions in our life in Chapter 1, right? So when you are asked about your learning style and how you adjust to new situations, you will know the answer. I like that!

These are two important issues to consider (now be honest with yourself):

1. How prepared do you feel you are since completing your education program?
2. Will the position you are considering provide you with the experience and support you need to function successfully as a new nurse?

If your answer to the first question is "not very prepared," you are not alone. If you waffle on your response to the second question, don't take the job. In fact, regardless of the nursing school you attended, new grads have a lot to learn.

Maria writes,

*Oh crap, I think I need to start nursing school all over again—the academic part, where I was supposed to learn something. I remember going to school all those long days and studying for all those tedious exams, but all of that information has decided to no longer come forward in my brain or when it comes, I am always afraid I am wrong.*

*Each day that I am on the PICU (pediatric intensive care unit) I realize how much I really don't know. I can take vitals like nobody's business. Oh and those pesky beeping IV (intravenous) machines, I can make them stop. But you want to put me in charge of monitoring someone's life and health? Are you serious? I am so afraid that I am going to be in a patient's room as they go into cardiac arrest and I am going to be a moron that runs out to my preceptor and says, "Umm, my patient isn't breathing and he no longer has a pulse. Do you think I should start CPR (cardiopulmonary resuscitation)?" God, I hope if something like that does happen I'll react the way I was taught. I used to think I was that person who could handle the situation, but now I have been humbled. OK, maybe I will do CPR, but what about all the signs before that? Will I pick up on those?*

*I think I just need to take a breath and realize that I am not supposed to know everything right now—learning is what I am supposed to be doing here.*

Learning is the focus of your first few weeks, months, and years. That is the good part about being a nurse; there is always something new to learn. Every grad feels like she could have used much more clinical in school. In our *First Year Study* we frequently heard:

"We needed more med-surg." or

"No, I don't need more med/surg, I should have gone right into mental health (or another specialty), which is what I was most interested in." and

"The whole process of entering nursing is overwhelming but start by doing small things."

Bird by bird, buddy. That is the advice from those who went before you.

Alena reflects back on her first-year experience and wants you to know this:

*There's a big learning curve when you get your first job. At least 15 people will tell you this when you start working. What they don't tell you is that the information you acquire in nursing school is a small portion of what you should know, and you have some catching up to do. The solid education, on which nurses rely to save lives, is the most important groundwork of their career. But that is not the only thing that makes a nurse. I have learned that great nurses are not born; they must be nurtured and developed. While they should already have an intrinsic reserve of patience and respect for human beings, these characteristics alone do not save lives nor do they keep patients safe. Drive and the ability to learn quickly are essential.*

So where do you start the journey? The old adage was "Get a year of med-surg under your belt." In many facilities, the year of adult med-surg is no longer required. Right now there are some specialty areas that offer meticulously designed orientations just for the new grad. Other specialty units still say they will only accept nurses with some experience under their belt.

Melissa, after 1 year out of school as a successful new grad, has some sage advice for students in their senior year:

*I know now more than ever that being a medical-surgical floor nurse is not my true passion, and I find myself eagerly awaiting my 1-year anniversary which opens the opportunity to bid on any other job in the hospital. When I was applying for jobs, I was adamantly discouraged by many nurses, nursing professors, and nurse recruiters from applying for a labor and delivery or maternal/child nursing position under the long-held belief that a new nurse must first "pay her dues" as a medical-surgical nurse before choosing a "specialty." In my senior year, for my senior nursing internship when I was working in LDRP (labor, delivery, recovery, postpartum), I felt that I could really become an expert at it. I was passionate, excited, eager, and idealistic. I was energized by the autonomy and patient-teaching opportunities. And most importantly, I was excited to go into work for every shift.*

*Unfortunately, I do not feel the same way about my current job as a float nurse. I have kept in touch with many of my classmates, and what I do see are many of my fellow students excelling as nurses in specialties that they are very passionate about: ICU, pediatric cardiology, NICU, ER (emergency room). If I could do it all over again I wouldn't necessarily give up my float pool experiences because I have learned so much about organization, prioritization, and the adult and geriatric populations that I know will serve me well as any type of nurse; but I wouldn't necessarily recommend it to other nursing students either.*

Liz went right into a specialty in a large urban hospital:

*I was told to start in med-surg, but I knew that was not going to make me happy. So I called human resources and told them I wanted to work in L & D and they laughed at me. I called the nurse manager five times, e-mailed her, and finally just showed up. She said she'd give me a shot.*

*I'll tell you, all the skills I worried about, I learned very quickly. What is important is critical thinking: Why is this happening? Talk to others, doctors, CNAs, nurses, so you can figure out what is going on, and you'll be fine.*

When you are considering a position, you need to make sure your new job offers you the support and information you need to function as a new nurse. Amanda said that on her interview they told her to consider the first year of nursing as her fifth year in school because you would be learning so much and would have many to support her learning. That is what you are looking for too! But first (drum roll please), the ever-looming NCLEX.

After graduation, when the celebrations die down, the studying really begins. The first hurdle in your postgrad life is to pass the NCLEX exam. The NCLEX is a portal one must pass through to enter nursing. Passing the exam does not necessarily mean you will be a good nurse. But you must pass the exam to be able to practice as a nurse. There are many good CDs, books, online and in-person classes out there (see Appendix). No matter what approach you choose to study, the key to the exam is to practice, practice, practice. You are the only one who can decide what the best way is for you to practice for the exam.

- Can you make yourself review the 3,500 CD questions daily?
- Or, is it better to buy the review series and answer questions in a specific clinical area and then go back and review the topic?
- Or, is your time and money well spent on a review course?

You know how you learn best, so choose what works for you and stick to it. Tori writes,

*I graduated. I celebrated. I still have to study? I couldn't quite wrap my head around this concept. I was so excited to have closed another chapter in my life and to begin writing a new one, except I forgot that this chapter has a twist. I still have to take the NCLEX (National Council Licensure Examination). I now have a diploma but I've yet to take the mother of all final exams.*

*I made a conscious decision to take time off between graduation and New Years. That meant no NCLEX 3500, no Saunders, no worrying about the exam. I also made the decision not to begin working until I passed the test—the less pressure the better. I enjoyed the holidays, spent time with friends I hadn't seen since I began the nursing program, and reveled in the fact that I was one step closer to a paycheck.*

*On January 2, I became a studying machine, and 100 study questions a day was my goal. I'd heard a rumor that the more practice questions, the better. So*

*100 questions a day multiplied by at least 2¹/₂ months before I'd take the test equaled more questions than I could count on my fingers and toes—a good sign I figured. The questions were tedious, and I often thought that what I was doing was ridiculous yet maybe not enough, but because I'm not much for reading information from textbooks, my studying had to be focused on questions and learning from wrong answers.*

*On my first interview, the nurse recruiter said it was preferred that new grads start after passing the NCLEX. At least we were on the same page.*

*It's now the middle of March. I have a job and no test date, and now I'm starting to get antsy. Most of the people I keep in contact with from my graduating class have passed the NCLEX. The two girls I was closest with during school also passed, so I was really beginning to feel the pressure. I started thinking to myself, well, someone has to fail, why not me? Then I began thinking about how I should've started work so I wouldn't feel so out of practice and it'd keep my mind off the test. It was at this time I became discouraged and nervous because I hadn't heard anything from the New York State Board of Nursing and they had my paperwork for the past 6 weeks. Also, I'd been studying for almost 10 weeks, and I was getting pretty sick of it. I found myself fantasizing about throwing my Saunders book into a fire or putting the NCLEX 3500 CD through my mom's paper shredder twice, just to make sure.*

*On the first day of the seventh week, I received my ATT (Authorization to Take the Test) by e-mail and set my test date for a week later, the earliest appointment I could get. I didn't mess around with my study schedule and thought positively all week. I also didn't tell anyone except for my parents, brothers, and non-nursing best friend that I was taking it. The less people who knew meant the less people I may have to tell I didn't pass.*

*Not much to say about test day except that I arrived half an hour early for my 8 a.m. appointment despite being out until after midnight the night before because I went to a concert (I did this on purpose. If I didn't do something good to tire me out, I would've been up all night worrying about the test.). I took a number and waited until they called me into the testing room that houses about 20 computer stations. I was first in the room and began my test alone. The first question I narrowed down to two answers that I swore were right and said to myself, if this is how the entire test is going to be I'm definitely up the creek without a paddle.*

*Throughout the test, there were questions on illnesses and drugs that I'd never heard of, but I kept telling myself that it was OK and if I stayed positive, that I'd do well. I answered question 170, and the computer decided it was time to end my 2½ months of worry and wonder (I took the actual test for 2 hours). I walked out to my car and blasted the radio the entire way home. I was finished.*

*I lied. I wasn't finished. The waiting-to-see-if-you-passed-or-failed part is the absolute worst part of the NCLEX. I had to wait 2 business days to get my unofficial results, but I began checking the Pearson Web site about an hour after I got home. I tested on Thursday and keeled over at the thought of having to wait until Monday to get my results. I never did know if Saturday counted as a business day. Thursday and Friday went pretty much the same. I stayed in my pajamas, watched TV, and ate ice cream straight from the carton. I didn't want to know anybody at this point and vice versa. I had convinced myself that I hadn't passed and I'd need to retake the test. I thought if I convinced myself now it wouldn't come as such a shock when I got my grade. Saturday morning at about 10:30 I checked the Web site again and my grade was up for my viewing pleasure. I crossed every appendage I have and clicked the link. The page stated my name, a few ID numbers, and my grade. Pass. I can't remember a time when I jumped so high or screamed so loud—maybe in third grade when New Kids on the Block came to town. I ran into the living room and hugged my mom, I called my dad who was out to breakfast, and I text-messaged my brothers, one of whom who was vacationing in Las Vegas (nice life, huh?). I was so relieved. My hard work had truly paid off. I had completed this chapter in my life. I could start my job with the confidence I'd need to make it through my first year. My new chapter could finally begin.*

*So what had I learned from the past 2½ months?*

- *I learned that studying over time is way better than cramming it in, as evidenced by my 100-questions-a-day method.*
- *I learned that you'll just know if a job and a hospital are right for you.*
- *I learned that staying positive will help you get through the crummy times, and that eating ice cream out of a carton will not—and has a 3-pound consequence.*
- *And finally, I learned that Saturday is a business day.*

What a great description of reality nursing! The test, the job, a break. Think about how you want to manage the start of your new career. Sarah took a break from school first and then took the NCLEX exam. You may be able to tell by her tone:

*I had passed the NCLEX. I could not believe it. I did not take a course; that was too much money.*

*I got a book and studied the questions. I made a list of what I did not know but never went back to it.*

*I followed my gut, figured if I did not pass, so be it. During the day of the test I tried to be present. I took a quiet minute before I started and just focused on each question. I decided if I got to 75 and it did not stop, I'd get some water, walk around, and come back and keep going.*

You will pass the NCLEX. You just have to figure out which style of studying works for you. If you do not pass the first time, go back to your school and find out what they recommend to help you be better prepared for the next time. They want you to succeed too, so go ahead and make an appointment with your faculty. You would not be the first person not to pass the first time. Don't let your ego get in your way of preparing for your next try. Go ahead and make an appointment with your faculty to design an individualized study plan. We need you in nursing!

# Job Search

Some new grads look for jobs before taking the NCLEX; others take the time to prepare for the exam, pass, and then take a break to regroup so they can approach the job search with new energy. Then again, some students are hired before they graduate.

Monica chose to stay on the unit where she had her senior internship:

*I feel so at home on my own unit. It was such a valuable mix of opportunities to have done the senior internship, then the CNA stint and now moving into the RN role. My comfort is so enhanced just from knowing my surroundings and my coworkers.*

The last sentence should be emphasized. Knowing the surroundings and your coworkers is huge. Knowing where to park is major! In any new job there should be opportunities to become familiar with the physical environment with helpful responses when you ask where the dirty utility is, not the "how can you not know that?" look. If you have a senior internship you will get an inside view of the work environment. This may lead you to want to sign on immediately or move on as fast as possible. We have students competing for internships in the ICUs and the ED, the cool places.

One mature, second bachelor's student did very well in her ICU internship, but in reflecting on the experience, recognized that as a new nurse, she needed to work with some patients who were going to get well and walk out. She decided that for a new nurse the ICU had too many deaths after giving so much care.

Pay attention to your response to your final internship or senior capstone experience. Seeing people in pain, watching patients struggle with their illness and, being asked to provide comfort measures are challenging experiences for any nurse. You need time to process your reactions to the vulnerability that your patients and you will experience. Take time to share your reactions with other new nurses, and find a way to manage this awesome responsibility in your own life so you can come back the next day and give the care your patients need. Pay attention to the effect that caring so deeply has on you. Talk to peers and friends who will actively listen to everything you have to say. There are facilities that provide support groups for nurses to process their feelings about their new job. Although you will be inordinately busy in your new position, make time to attend new nurse meetings. Talking with peers will help you to feel not so alone with your emotions and your fears. You will feel better knowing others have had similar experiences and will come back refreshed or at least better prepared to take care of your next patient.

There needs to be a balance between the patient's needs, the organization's requirements, and your own health. Consider daily journaling so you can get some of those thoughts and feelings out of your head and your body (we all hold stress in different parts of our body; where does your stress show up?) Learning how to manage the incredible responsibility of being a nurse takes many forms, from talking to peers, to journal writing, exercising, laughing, and playing. Find what works for you. Personally, I need them all! Take care of yourself so you can care for others.

Begin by taking time to reflect on what you bring to the job and what you need to learn. Being self-aware is essential in nursing. You have an opportunity to practice skills and gain information in orientation. The more aware you are of your learning style and what you need to practice, the more successful you will be. Before you know it, you'll be assigned your own patients.

As a new nurse observed,

*The thing about nursing that I feel is different from most other "out-of college jobs" is that there is no entry position. I am working right next to these senior nurses and we are expected to do the same things, at the same pace, and with the same excellence. This creates a lot of pressure. It also creates a great sense of accomplishment knowing that I am a "nurse"; a real live one.*

There will always be jobs for nurses. The first position just may not be your dream job. You may have to start in long-term care or a rehabilitation facility. Both offer many opportunities to work closely with patients and their families, improve your skills, and expand your knowledge base. Whether acute care, long-term care, or rehab, you should still look for a unit that supports new grads. They need you too.

## Are You Attracted to a Magnet?

As you are choosing hospitals to apply to, consider what a magnet facility has to offer. But before the interview, do some homework on what the magnet process is all about so you will be well versed in the magnet philosophy for your interview. Here's a thumbnail sketch of the magnet story: The term *magnet* is used to indicate that selected hospitals have the reputation and work environment that attracts and retains nurses. A hospital with a magnet designation means the American Nurses Credentialing Center (ANCC) has given the facility the official magnet designation in recognition of the excellent nursing work environment, the innovations in nursing care, and the high quality of patient care. In a national survey, over 20 years ago, 41 hospitals were nominated by their own staff as great places for nurses to work. The administration and staff in each facility were interviewed to learn about the strengths in the work environment. At that time 14 forces of magnetism were identified. Recently, these forces have been consolidated into five forces of magnetism:

- Transformational leadership
- Structural empowerment
- Exemplary professional nursing practice
- New nursing knowledge
- New nursing innovations (Wolf, Triolo, & Reid Ponte, 2008)

Evidence indicates magnet hospitals lead not only to recruitment and retention of nurses but improves patient outcomes (Aiken, Smith, & Lake,

1994). On your interview listen for how these forces of magnetism are described, or if you are interviewing at a facility that does not have a magnet designation, ask about these aspects of the work environment. The application for a magnet designation can be costly for a hospital, so they may well have many of the components of magnetism but are not an official magnet facility. In your interview, whether with a designated magnet facility or not, ask about these essential workplace qualities:

- Shared governance
- Certification and formal education
- Evidence-based practice and nursing research

Shared governance means the governance structure of nursing is shared between the staff and the administration. Decision making on nursing practice is not handed down from the top but rather decisions are made with consultation between staff and administration. The staff have input into practice decisions through unit-based nursing councils that meet with the administration. What this means for you, as a staff nurse, is that you are expected to identify ideas to improve patient care or to better the nursing work process. You have an active role in deciding how nursing is practiced. You are expected to be a leader. Don't be reticent in inquiring about what the nurse role is in governance. The governance structure influences how each nurse practices. Not only will you learn what is expected of you in your new role by asking such questions, but you will demonstrate your awareness of the nursing work environment and that will be impressive!

Every hospital claims they want their nurses to be leaders. Ask how this ideal is actually supported in practice. Is there leadership training? Leadership mentoring? Do they promote from within? Some places are proud to promote their own staff, while other hospitals believe they need to look for outside candidates for leadership positions. What is your facility's philosophy about leadership? Can you be promoted for clinical excellence? In the past, to be promoted, nurses had to leave the bedside and move into a management or education track. Today, advancement in nursing is different. You know as well as I do, with the acuity and complexity of patient care, we need leaders at the bedside. Thus, clinical ladder programs were created so that the bedside nurses can move from clinical nurse 1 to 2 to 3, and so on (see Chapter 10 to learn more about clinical ladders). Some facilities require specialty certification to be promoted up the ladder. Make sure to learn about the process required to obtain specialty certification and the reimbursement policy for formal education during the interview process. An important nursing value is lifelong education. Nurses are expected to continue their education. The ANA Code of Ethics states: "The nurse owes the same duties to self and others, including the responsibility to preserve integrity and safety, to maintain competence and continue personal and professional growth" (American Nurses Association, 2001). Each state requires a certain amount of hours per year be devoted to continuing education. Ask about continuing education opportunities and tuition reimbursement policies. With ongoing education being a central component of our Code of Ethics, asking does not look pushy, it looks professional. Trust me.

In magnet facilities, staff nurses collaborate on developing evidence to support their suggestions to improve patient care through the academic literature. Staff is involved at all levels of decision making in assessing and implementing innovations. Magnet facilities are exciting places to work. The mood, enthusiasm, and collegiality are palpable in magnet hospitals. Consider a magnet facility as a place to look for a job.

## You're Hired!

Congratulations! You got the job you were hoping for.

Tori writes,

*When I was studying for the NCLEX I began going to the open house programs that hospitals hold and I went on a few interviews. I focused my job search on university-affiliated hospitals in New York City and still managed to have more than my fair share of options. I chose a medical floor at NYU Medical Center, and they chose me too. I never thought I'd walk into a hospital and know I belonged there, but this place screamed TORI. They offered a 12-month new graduate residency program, 8 weeks of preceptor work, and another 6 to 8 weeks of additional training on the day shift, if necessary. They weren't into pushing me right into the 8 p.m. to 8 a.m. shift that I'd eventually be working, which I also appreciated. They encouraged further education and advanced degrees. And I loved the fact they were willing to work with me on my start date.*

From the first interview on, Tori knew she had found a fit. This update just in:

*I can hardly believe it was 2 years ago. I had a hard but enjoyable run at NYU Medical Center for a year and a half. They have some of the best nurses around. I learned so much from them and really worked on my critical thinking skills. I left that position in September and have since been working in an office-based endoscopy suite, so I'm gaining PACU experience and getting lots of interaction with patients, which I love!*

If you wondering if the fit between you and the position you are interviewing for will be as clear to you as it was to Tori, I'd say, "Yes, if the job is a good match, you will know." If you are not feeling it, pay attention to what that means.

So, you are ready to start your first position. What can you expect in orientation? Most hospitals have general classes that everyone is required to attend and is followed by unit-specific classes. Next you are sent off to the particular unit with a preceptor that was hand-chosen to match your needs. Some places are recognizing all the classes upfront are TMI (too much information) for the new grad so they are spreading the information out over months so the new nurse can be in classes and also have hands-on clinical experience.

Lauren writes about her first week:

*I made it through my first week of orientation. Now comes the hard part— making it through my first day on the floor. It still hadn't hit me yet that I was a nurse, I forgot. I think it hit me when they asked all the nurses in the room to raise their hand . . . it took me a second to realize I was included in that because I'm not a student nurse anymore. Many times I felt proud during this week to be a nurse and say yes, I am a nurse; but absolutely terrified because I am a nurse. I can't say that I'm a student now and put it on to someone else because I am the person to have the answers.*

*I do know that I'll be glad to be working 12-hour shifts; doing the 8-hour days 5 days a week is not for me. I think I will enjoy my days off during the week.*

*I finally got to meet my preceptor on Friday. That in itself is nerve wracking. What if we don't get along? Or she thinks I'm incompetent? I feel like I'm back in the student role all over again, with the nerves and desire to do well and get things right and learn. I just hope I didn't forget everything in the past few months of not doing it. Everyone keeps saying, "you'll be fine," but they don't know that, and it's frustrating to hear. I'm sure I'll make it through the day, but I'm still scared. I feel like I'm going back to my first clinical rotation all over again with all those unknowns.*

Remember, this is a journey that you are going to take one day at a time, bird by bird. Sarah's description of orientation was a little different from the usual. Her orientation was the beginning of the year-long residency program. So the residency orientation was a time when the staff educators really focused on how to help their orientees manage the stress of a new job and for many, a new town.

Sarah reported,

*The social experience was fabulous. We were 25 new grads from all over the country. They really encouraged us to get to know each other with the mantra "be kind to your peers." So we planned a rafting trip together. That was a blast!*

Whether you are in a residency or not, being with other new grads is key. Lauren recognized this in her first week:

*There is another new grad starting at the same time as me, so I did feel happy about that. I don't want to be the only one going through orientation. I also found out that there is another new grad who started about a month ago, so in reality there are three of us. What a relief!*

Damien had been an LPN before coming back to school but during orientation she too felt overwhelmed by the new responsibility:

*It was not until starting orientation at AMC that I really began to appreciate how little I knew about nursing, and what a difficult road still lies ahead. When I arrived "on the floor," I felt like a new student on the first day of clinical. Nearly every time I showed up for a new shift, this feeling of "overwhelm" would arise. By the time orientation was officially finished, this sensation of utter insecurity had gradually begun to subside and to be replaced with bits of discombobulated knowledge.*

This is not to overwhelm you but to let you know that the feelings of being unprepared, knowing nothing, and being on your own for the first time are common and actually what you should expect. Nurses say they'd actually worry if the new grad was too confident and did not ask questions. As my friend Martha said, "Questions from the new nurse are the safety net between the knowledge a new nurse brings and keeping the patient safe."

Sarah T. was offered a position on the unit where she did her senior internship, which lessened the anxiety of starting in an unfamiliar environment. In her last days of orientation she reflected,

*Three days of orientation left. This week was a transition time. It began with a workshop I participated in for new grad nurses called Simulated Bedside Emergencies for the New Nurse. My CNS [clinical nurse specialist] suggested I go. There were other new nurses with varying degrees of practice experience. It was a very helpful review of emergency procedures: the code cart, the role of the various people in a code, and then how to simulate a code. The important part for me was the simulation of a code at the end with a SimMan, just like I had used in our school lab. Afterward, we sat down with the instructors to debrief and watch ourselves on video. They first asked what our impression was. I said I felt that it was a little chaotic and I didn't feel like we had a leader. Then we watched the video. Two minutes in, it became obvious that in fact, I had been leading the code until the code team arrived. They say someone always ends up taking the lead. It was a little embarrassing to realize that I had no idea, no ability to see from the outside what role I had played. But I was encouraged by the instructor's positive responses to my actions, saying I had done a good job and in fact we had all done a good job and worked very well together as a team.*

*This was a powerful experience for me. I left feeling good and I thought about what had happened and my reaction for several days afterward. Here is some of what I realized: (1) every birth is an emergency (and I work in L&D); (2) I was one of the oldest new grads there, with 4 years of non-nursing medical field experience, and I have more life experience than some new nurses (having come to nursing as a second career), which does in fact count for something! and (3) I have learned a lot during these past 3 months. The timing was also really good for me. I felt good about my ability to lead this particular simulated code. It gave me a needed self-esteem boost. In the days that followed, it sunk in that I am about to take on a lot of responsibility.*

*During the several weeks before this workshop, I had begun to get a little freaked out about coming off orientation, confiding to my close friends that I wasn't sure I would be ready to be on my own after Thanksgiving; I wasn't sure I would have time to experience all the things I needed to be comfortable on the floor. My friends all reassured me, saying they had confidence that I was up for the challenge. I told myself they actually had no idea, none of them having experienced what I was going through or really knowing what was expected of me. I doubted myself. But this SIM code helped put things in perspective. It gave me some confidence, and it helped me realize that this is just how it works. No one ever feels totally comfortable when they have their first day on the floor. There is no way to experience every possible scenario. Even the experienced nurses learn new things all the time and ask for help. The nurses on my floor have told me time and again that they will be there to support me as a new nurse, and not only that, they have already proved it and begun that process. Most importantly, I realized I had to start owning my nursing practice, really for the first time. Even if I don't always feel like I can do it, I needed to start acting like I can. I have always aimed to do this with my patients, knowing they need to feel secure with their nurse; but it is more challenging to do this with my colleagues, other nurses, and the doctors. Now is the time to step up, to become an L&D nurse with everyone in my life, to make this role my own.*

It is a gradual journey, this learning to be a nurse. As Sarah observed, "Sometimes we don't even recognize our own growth." The first few weeks are intense. During this transition it is very important to be kind to yourself. Keep in touch with your school friends, be open to making new friends, let your family know how you are doing, and find routines of comfort whether it be regular exercise, a massage, journaling, meditation, or a night out.

Maria reflects back on her first year:

*I knew that I was there to learn and become part of this team, but there is so much more involved in this process—things you never even realized. I really believe that the first year out can really make or break a person. I say that only because of the emotional aspect that is involved in being a novice nurse—especially an overachieving, self critical, self-doubting, new nurse.*

Maria captures the spirit of most new nurses: overachieving, being self-critical and self-doubting. Be gentle with yourself. The expectations of others are enough without adding your own self-critical voice. How do you take care of yourself? Build in a routine. Find the time. Integrate self-care into your life. It is not an add-on. Your own routine needs to be central to your well-being. This is a lesson you will be preaching to many patients due to the fact that at least 80% of modern-day illness is stress related. So be sure to listen to such wise advice for yourself. If you needed a nurse, you would want that individual to be well rested, focused, attentive, and present. Be that nurse. Start now. OK, I am getting off my self-care soapbox. You get the idea.

## On Your Own!

By 6 weeks, orientation is ending and you are placed on the shift that you will work. You will have moved from a precepted experience to being a real nurse. Although it feels like you are on your own, you are not, really. The other nurses are invested in your succeeding. You will begin to notice a hint of confidence, an increased ability to know how to ask questions, and actually feel like you have chosen the right place to work.

Damien recognized,

*My preceptors have been the most important people in my professional develop-ment this year. I worked with two individuals, both very knowledgeable, each with her own unique style and manner of teaching. The first, J., was very young but mature and experienced to a surprising degree. We worked together for about 6 weeks doing 12-hour day shifts. The relationship has been very much like that of a kindly master to an apprentice. J. was able to gently guide me through the basics of PICU care, to point out the essentials of hospital policy, and to generally prepare me for my transition to the night shift and the second half of my orientation.*

*K. was my second preceptor. She is smart, almost to a fault. There is practically nothing that she doesn't know about PICU, and she is proud of it. I would com-pare this relationship to one of a benevolent drill sergeant preparing a recruit for the battlefield. Many times I wished I had chosen a different path and was filled with anxiety before arriving at the start of each new shift. Perseverance eventu-ally prevailed, and I "graduated" on to being allowed to work independently.*

*Luckily, the assignments I was given at 6 weeks were not overly demanding, and there were always resource people around who could answer questions and lend a hand. Gradually, this whole experience, everything from the prerequi-sites I took more than 6 years ago, nursing school, working as an LPN, and the training at AMC, all seem to be somehow miraculously rearranging them-selves into a working model. Feelings of apprehension are slowly being sup-planted by ability and confidence.*

That is the good news. By 6 weeks your education, your review of skills during orientation, and your time on the unit are all coming together.

A new nurse reflected,

*So, I've been working in this career now for 7 weeks, 6 of which have been on the floor. Seven weeks is such a small amount of time in the midst of the other nurses who have been working for 20 to 30 years. I have had many other nurses that I work with call me the "baby" on the floor. It is very endearing, and I do feel like I am just beginning to "crawl" when they are running, jumping, and maneuvering their way through the day. Like anything else in life, everything comes in due time, and someday soon I will be walking on my own with them to guide me.*

*The worry I feel sometimes is that this moment when I have to be on my own is coming soon, in 5 weeks to be exact. It is strange, however, because some days when things go smoothly I feel like I am really doing this on my own and it feels so good. It actually feels surreal. And then BAM, something or someone puts me back in my place. It is a godsend that this happens, however, because it keeps me in check, keeps me asking questions, and keeps me from feeling like I should know everything because I shouldn't. Remember, I am the "baby," and babies need to ask questions to learn and need guidance in order to grow.*

Your team is there for you: your supervisor, manager, resource nurse, and the other staff nurses. They are there for each other. There are resources on the computer and in other departments like the physicians, the chaplain, the social worker, or the ethics nurse. Health care changes so fast that you will be learning your whole career. All nurses attend clinical updates regularly. You'd certainly want the nurse working with your mother or son to have the latest information, wouldn't you? This is one of the exciting aspects of nursing, the research being done, the new evidence available, updates to attend.

Lisa reminds us,

*No matter how much time spent doing clinical while in school, or even spent in a preceptorship, you're not going to be able to see everything, it's luck of the draw—what patient happens to be in the bed at that time. It is not realistic to be able to experience everything before you start your first job. I think it is important to be given the time to take all those steps so you can operate in a safe way. Use your resources. There are a fair amount of resources on the computer. Use the nursing supervisor.*

*I had a patient say her heart felt racy, the patient was in v-tach (ventricular tachycardia). Coincidently, the nursing supervisor called to ask a question. I said, "I'm a fairly new nurse; my patient is in v-tach." The night nurses had gone to dinner, so not a lot of people were on the floor. The nursing supervisor sent the rapid response team. The team told me what to do: "Stand in the corner. Write down vital signs." Just then the doctors happened to walk in to see the other patient in the room and asked if we needed help. They ended up placing a central line in the patient.*

*Afterward I felt completely numb. An hour later, I started to cry. I came home, took a hot shower, had a cup of tea. Again, in testament to the exceptional place at which I work, the nurses called and just wanted to check and see how I was doing. They said, "This didn't happen because of what you did. You did everything right. Everything you could have done, you did." I thought that was really exceptional. Where else does anyone take that time? They were kind and considerate. This is what makes it such a nice place to work.*

You will always be learning. Nursing is humbling in that way.

D'arcy reflects,

*I kind of know what I'm doing, but then I don't know what I'm doing again. Everyone seems to tell to me that's just how nursing is. There will always be something presented to you that you haven't seen before, even if you've been there 25 years. It is constantly changing. And if you don't change and you're not constantly learning, then you're out of date!*

The other nurses, your friends from school, and your family can all provide support during this time of transition. For some new nurses, the introduction to nursing is more difficult than it should be. Follow these helpful tips:

1. Pay attention to how you feel.
2. Don't isolate yourself.
3. Stay in touch with other new grads for support.

Tina shares,

*I had a preceptor who did everything with me at first. She was very willing to answer questions and was supportive. Unfortunately, after 2 months, she told me I should be handling a full load by myself. And, after that she only told me what I was doing wrong or doing too slowly. She did not give me any encouragement. I was beside myself, wondering why I EVER chose to become a nurse. I was sure I would never cut it as a nurse and especially as an ED (emergency department) nurse. Some of the other nurses must have seen my dismay because a few started coming forth and encouraging me on the sly. Thank goodness for them because that is one of the things that kept me going. My husband, children, and mother were the others who kept me going. They had complete faith in me and were actually disgusted that I was so down on myself. Of COURSE you can do it, they'd reply when I would voice my doubts. So I kept showing up for work, driving there with knots in my stomach, and tightness in my chest all the way. I spent the whole shift feeling that way, too. I'd sweat, my hands shook, and I was terrified almost the whole time. The smell of the Pyxis (med dispensing machine) would give me chest pain. I was so scared to give meds, especially IV meds. I felt like an impostor. I wasn't a nurse. I felt like a fraud telling my patients I was a nurse. It took a long time for me to say, "Hi, I'm Tina and I'll be YOUR nurse." That sounded too committed. I felt safer saying, "Hi, I'm Tina, one of the nurses." Anyway, the bottom line is that it was awful in the beginning. If it wasn't for the investment of 4 years in college, the paycheck we needed so badly, the health insurance we also needed, and my pride (how could I face all my family and friends to tell them I couldn't handle being a nurse?!), I would have quit in a heartbeat. I would say to myself, "I hate nursing, I hate this place, I hate this job." Somehow, it made me feel better to say it to myself.*

*The good news is, eventually, one shift at a time, it just got better and better. And I got a new preceptor who just kept telling me I was doing great all the time. That helped me so much, it was what I needed so badly.*

"I had a preceptor that kept telling me I was doing a great job." That is what you should be hearing too. If you are not, consult with your nurse manager. The organization has invested time and money in you. They want you to succeed. You are not in this alone. You have a whole team behind you, and you should feel that way. The culture you work in should support the journey of the new nurse. You want to look forward to going to work every day. Nursing can be a difficult job. The team you work with is critical to your success; the relationship between nurses, physicians, and other colleagues can make or break your experience. Put yourself in a place consciously designed to support your success so you can be the nurse you dreamed of and the nurse the patients need.

Alena, an excellent nurse, reports it is not a direct route from school into practice. She reinforces that the first year is a journey with pit stops and side detours that will eventually lead to your destination:

*When I started at Oregon's largest level-one trauma center, I was a world away from the elderly patients with urinary tract infections who lie in the 10-bed ICU in rural Massachusetts. The 20-bed cardiac surgical unit was chaos. Open hearts, sepsis, and the lateral transfers from other ICUs were shocking. I desperately searched my brain for anything to bring light to the patients' conditions. Yet I had nearly nothing. These were the sickest patients I had ever seen. They had tubes, pumps, and drains attached to them and I couldn't pronounce let alone know how they worked. Although I completed the coursework of the hospital internship program, I was quickly told I didn't have enough experience to make it as a nurse on the unit. For 3 months I was sent to gain experience on an abdominal transplant acute care ward. Being a proud new graduate, I was disheartened, defeated, and embarrassed. I was a failure at something I had worked so hard for.*

*On the floor I learned the hallmark skills of nursing: to organization therapeutic communication, and to run my butt off. I learned that to break the 4 p.m. wall I needed my second cup of coffee to limp to the change of shift. I came to understand that working on the floor was as hard, if not harder, than working in the ICU. In about 3 months I was ready to come back to the unit, repeating the 3-month internship.*

*Today I am certified in CVVH (continuous veno-venous hemofiltration), open heart recovery, and ventricular assist devices. I am certified to use and teach the use of PiCCO technology. I am a preceptor, mentor, American Association of Critical Care Nurses (AACN) member, and proud certified critical care nurse (CCRN). The cardiac surgical ICU is now my home where I am most comfortable, where my second family is. It is here that I exercise my autonomy and prepare for emergency situations that have yet to present themselves. I am not afraid to question resident's jejune orders and collaborate with attendings. I have participated in multiple critical care conferences, seminars, and morbidity and mortality conferences (M+Ms) to increase my awareness of issues in critical care medicine.*

*But my education progresses each day I show up for work, coffee in hand. I learn by people explaining to me, yelling at me, and questioning my judgment. I learn by defending my judgment. New nurses and new doctors are taught the same way. We are thrown into situations, mistakes are made, and we learn from them. Often it is hard to ask questions of (a) people you don't know and (b) people who aren't friendly. Ask anyway. Pay attention to the hesitation you feel about a specious order. Don't be afraid to go above a resident's head and ask their attending for clarification. Page at 3 a.m. if you must. Always remember the five rights of medication management. Above all else, keep your patients safe.*

*The beginning of my career was focused around learning about the ICU process and transitioning to appliance management. Orienting to open hearts, VADs (ventricular assist devices), CVVH, and balloon pumps was rewarding and challenging. I earned my ICU stripes one complex patient at a time. Feeling comfortable with the level-one trauma and crashing patients has become part of my everyday life. A patient is no longer "a good learning experience." Instead, most often they are another sad case. I am not afraid to admit the ICU intimidates me and saddens me every day. It is now in my career that I'm more focused on the patients and their families. I make every attempt to connect with bodies that are intubated and sedated. As a nurse, I'm able to heal in different ways than medicine. I have the ability and time to give a personal touch, connect with people on an intimate level while having the textbook knowledge to save a life. I make every attempt to explain to patients and families the difficult road to recovery. For the untrained eye, I try to bring order to an environment that I once perceived as chaos.*

This is the story, right from the front line.

## FINAL WORDS

These poignant observations are from a first-year nurse who has just been through what you are about to do:

*New nurses need to be willing to learn, hear criticism and advice from their peers. They need to respect patients and listen to them. Most of all, they need to have confidence in themselves and not beat themselves up for being slow and clumsy.*

*Skills . . . ahhh skills—the thing I worried most about and that is one of the least important things because they just come. You just develop them by doing. First, you watch, then you do with supervision, then you do it on your own. I stressed so much about skills in the beginning. I think we all did. New nurses need the ability to:*

- *Ask questions and look up information.*
- *Practice time management.*
- *Build self-confidence but not overconfidence.*

- *Develop communication skills to be able to talk to doctors and other nurses and patients.*
- *Prioritize patient needs.*
- *Develop knowledge of medications that will be used frequently in your area of practice.*
- *Listen to patients.*
- *Find someone to listen to you.*

*The new nurse should attempt to leave preconceptions and prejudices at home and practice with the attitude that every moment is a wonderful opportunity to learn, to grow, and to help another human being in need.*

# CONCLUSION

The expectations are high, the work is critical, and you will have an incredibly important role in our health-care system. My mentor Joyce Clifford said, "Nurses are like precious jewels," and I wholeheartedly agree with her. Your nursing care will have a ripple effect, from influencing the health of one patient to the health of the nation and our international community. You will be on the inside, in a position to know what works and what does not. You are entering nursing just at the right time, when nurses are publicly recognized as valuable and at the hub of the wheel of the health-care team. Never underestimate your influence. Work in a place that appreciates your unique contributions.

You have been through a rigorous educational program, passed the major licensing exam (that you will never have to take again!), and survived orienting to your first position. This is a journey. Choose the right path carefully so both you and your patients will benefit from this exciting adventure!

## References

Aiken, L., Smith, H., & Lake, E. (1994). Lower medicine mortality among a set of hospitals known for good patient care. *Medical Care. 32*(8), 771–787.

American Nurses Association (2001). Silver Springs, MD: Nursebooks.org

Lamott, A. (1994). *Bird by bird: Some instructions on writing and life.* New York: Pantheon.

Wolf, G., Triolo, P., & Reid Ponte, P. (2008). Magnet recognition program: The next generation. *Journal of Nursing Administration. 38*(4), 200–204.

# [CHAPTER 9]

# One Year Out

One year and still going strong! That will be *your* life. In fact, only after 9 months, Melissa said,

*I reached my ninth-month mark at Crouse Hospital and hence my ninth month as a working RN. And I have to say that when I look back to where I was only 9 months ago, I am extremely proud of how far I have come.*

In a year you will have accomplished an enormous amount. Let's look into the future so you can get a picture of where you are headed. What will it be like after you have worked as a nurse for a year? From the results of the *First Year Study* I can tell you that your feelings will be paradoxical. On one hand, you will feel like a pro with many skills and procedures under your belt. You will know how the floor works, who you can count on, and the personalities of your coworkers. On the other hand, you will realize how much there still is to learn.

"One year out and still learning" is how Melissa started her story. The nurses who have been practicing for a year report that they are confident in their abilities and recognize that they learn something new every day. After a year, the nurses report that they have moved from focusing solely on the list of tasks that need to be done to considering the whole patient and his or her family. They were starting to look beyond their particular unit-based responsibilities and become involved in hospital-wide committee work. Many of the nurses were considering moving to a new position, leaving the hospital for home care, or returning to graduate school.

Melissa, Tammi, Maria, and Neusa have very different positions, work different shifts, and come from different undergraduate programs. Melissa started in a float nurse position and has some sage advice to offer, Tammi went directly from school to working in the LDRP (labor, delivery, recovery,

147

postpartum) and was thrilled with the learning opportunities and teamwork she has experienced, Maria started on a patient-focused telemetry floor, but with staffing changes she is now considering a community position, and Neusa, who loves her job in pediatric oncology, is currently applying to graduate school. These four RNs exemplify the various career opportunities open to nurses, a distinct advantage of the nursing profession.

Melissa writes about her first year,

*I am still working as an evening medical-surgical float pool RN, which has continued to allow me to experience and learn from all areas of med-surg nursing including general medical, general surgical, cardiac/telemetry, hematology/oncology, gynecology, orthopedics, neurology, and even some emergency critical care. In the beginning I was oriented for 2 to 3 weeks on each floor, and every day I called the nursing supervisor an hour before my shift to see which floor I was being assigned to that night. I certainly feel that this job has allowed me to keep up many more skills and concepts that I would have otherwise lost had I taken a job on only one floor or in one specialty area. It has also been my experience at times that other more experienced nurses ask me for help with skills or patients that are "atypical" to their floor because they know I spend time on all floors. For example, the other day an orthopedic nurse with 20 years more experience than I asked me to assist her with accessing a patient's port-a-cath because I often do this on the oncology floor and patients with this type of central line rarely are admitted to her floor. Another time a seasoned cardiac nurse asked me to assist her with a patient with a PEG tube because I often take care of these patients on the general medical floor.*

*I am getting a lot of positive recognition for my work from my supervisor, colleagues, and patients. Many patients have told me that they are surprised to learn that I am a new graduate nurse because to them, my organization, efficiency, and knowledge base gives them the impression that I have been a nurse for a few years. These compliments and many other experiences have definitely helped boost my confidence and have provided me with the motivation to continue working every shift to my fullest potential instead of slipping into the very easy alternative of doing the minimum work necessary to make it through the night.*

*One of my main complaints is that as a float pool RN I do not get the benefit of having the same patient assignment each shift. I feel that this puts me at a disadvantage much of the time because I only get to see each of my patients for 8 hours or less, especially if I am floated to a different floor halfway through my shift. I feel that this often takes away much of my ability to make an educated nursing judgment about changes in a patient's condition or their plan of care: Are they more confused than yesterday? Does their wound look better or worse than yesterday? How are the family dynamics affecting this patient's condition or plan for discharge? Even the best shift-to-shift report or doctor's progress note cannot substitute for the relationships you form with patients when you take care of them for more than 1 day.*

Float nurses used to be the nurses who were very experienced and knew the hospital really well. Today, with the nursing shortage, float positions are no longer reserved for the experienced nurses.

Melissa accepted a float pool position right out of school. At first she oriented to all the units and then into her float position where she would work on a different unit every night. Being a float nurse from the start sounds exciting . . . and intimidating. Imagine being seen as an expert so early in your career? Yet Melissa's realistic assessment of her experience and her wish to know the trajectory of her patients, what they were like yesterday and where they will be tomorrow, makes sense. Because Melissa is floating to a different unit every shift, it may be time to move on to a different position and settle down on one unit. She says,

*What I do know is that I want to spend the rest of my career as a nurse and working in nursing, in whatever capacity that may be. I also know that at 23 and not yet a year out of school, I do not want to continue in a position that will lead to disillusionment and the loss of my ideals and passion for caring and learning. So I will wait until June when I can officially bid for a new position that will better suit me. Perhaps it will be LDRP, perhaps ICU, perhaps home care. Who knows? But it will be a position that I can completely immerse myself in and continue to learn and grow as a person and as a nurse. As we know, there are many alternative paths in nursing. That is the good news!*

A year on the job develops new ways of thinking, technical skills, and humility. Maria writes,

*One year out of school I realize that my thinking patterns have changed. I used to be three or four steps behind in my thinking in terms of patient care and organizing myself, and now I am only one or two steps behind—which is*

*great! I find so many things have become like second nature to me that 1 year ago scared the life out of me. My technical skills have improved so much and continue to do so. I have started to become involved in committees on my unit, I have a strong rapport with my attending physicians, and I could go on and on.*

Being involved in the committee work of nursing governance is so important for the patients. They need your new and fresh voice! You are on the front line; you know what isn't working and what needs to be changed. You do not need to wait 2 or 3 years to participate actively in the committee structure. In fact, if you do wait until you have been totally acclimated to the unit's ways of working, you will no longer have the outsider's perspective and may have lost the ability to see some of the issues that only a new nurse notices. It is never too soon to get involved. Also, active interest in your hospital and your professional organization helps to expand your view beyond your unit, provides you with a network of new colleagues, and can open your eyes to exciting career options.

Hospitals have active committees and councils where staff nurses discuss and debate policy issues affecting patient care. It is critical for the old guard to hear from the newer nurses with fresh eyes and opinions. But do so with sensitivity and respect for the traditional approach to getting things done. I took the less popular, more direct route in my first position. At 22 years old I was less than savvy in my new observation of old behavior. In the weekly staff meeting with psychiatrists, psychologists, social workers, nurses, and mental health counselors I blatantly asked, "Why do the nurses spend so much time in the nurses' station?" If looks could kill, it would have been curtains for me. A bit too direct, wouldn't you say? However, my less-than-delicately handled observation got the issue on the table and a conversation rolling that ultimately led to better patient care.

To improve quality care we need to hear from those who have not been acculturated into the old, accepted approaches. For example, recently a group of senior interns were commenting on the fact that staff nurses were reluctant to go into the rooms of patients who sustained injuries from attempting suicide. The seniors said that usually a sitter is assigned to these patients and the staff nurses stay away. It takes new eyes to notice these old habits. Here we have the most vulnerable patient, one who has attempted suicide, with the least skilled staff, a sitter. What is going on? This is a patient care problem that nursing needs to consider. This is a problem the new nurse can see, and by being involved in patient care committees, he or she can advocate for the most vulnerable. You do not have to be experienced to represent patient concerns and you do not have to wait to look out for your own concerns.

Maria brings up the tricky balance between all-consuming work and the rest of your life:

*All of these things have been challenging at times, and making it even more challenging is the fact that your home life still exists outside of the hectic work environment. Sometimes home can be your retreat from it all—you know how to do everything right at home and people are happy to see you. Or sometimes home can be another source of stress. We are all going through a struggle in one form or another. I think that it is very important to remember your mental health in the first year out of school. It can be very easy to get down on yourself. Always take time for yourself. It's important. When I had awful, horrible, miserable nights at work, I would always try to remember the feeling I had when I had a really wonderful night.*

Sounds like good advice to me! In Chapter 8 we talked about taking care of yourself. I believe a nurse is a role model for patients. Self-care is not an option but a requirement. New nurses have reported that balancing work and life is key to maintain. That balance is easy to get out of sync. To learn about your own work balance, draw a life pie periodically and see how you weigh in (Figure 9-1). There should be at least six equal slices of your life: friends and family, self-care, work, play, spirituality, and intellectual pursuits.

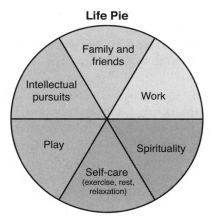

*Figure 9-1.* Life pie.

You can add other sections to the pie that represent your life. Then make each slice the size of the amount of time you are spending in that area. From the size of your life pie slices, are your work and life in balance?

In several recent studies, work/life balance has been cited as difficult for new nurses to manage. Pay attention to what works for you. Remember the four stages of role transition: honeymoon, shock/rejection, integration, and assimilation. From the time you accept a new job until your first few months at work you will be in the honeymoon stage "YES! I got a job as an RN!" Now that you have convinced the nurse manager that you are perfect for this job, you have to live up to your promise. Only too soon do you realize how much you still need to learn and the amount of responsibility that a nurse has. This realization signifies entry into the shock, and maybe, rejection stage, "Is this the right job for me?" or even some days, "Is this the right profession for me?" After about 6 months, you have your own patient assignment, pass your own meds, and some days feel like you can do this, actually feeling proud of your accomplishments. That is when you start to recover from the shock of what you have gotten yourself into and you begin to assimilate into the nurse's role. Along the way you begin to integrate your role as a nurse into the other roles in your life. You add nurse to being a son or daughter, uncle, aunt, sister, cousin, or friend.

From 6 to 12 months you are adjusting to the job expectations and how they fit with your life. Two 1-year survivors had very different approaches to managing work/life balance. Both nurses worked in cardiac care units (CCUs). Denise said that she worked as much overtime as possible and admitted it was exhausting, whereas Mark said he loved his job but never worked overtime because his job was so intense that when he left he needed to get away and recover. You can decide the balance of work and life that works best for you and strive to meet both your needs and the organization's needs. You won't be much good to the organization if you are unhappy. Pay attention to what is reasonable and what is unreasonable to ask of yourself.

Maria reported that she began on telemetry, and although she started on nights, she loved the patients and her coworkers. Then staffing problems hit and each nurse was assigned to one or two more patients than usual. The staffing shortage was supposed to be temporary, but next there were budget cuts. Maria did not feel like she could give the care her patients required, and the extra burdens of her role were wearing on her. When last we spoke she was debating how long she could manage the toll work was taking on her life. She was considering interviewing for a day clinic position. I encouraged her to look around and see what else was available so she could make an informed decision about whether to stay in a job that was familiar or move on to something new.

Neusa loved her job. She had been trained in a specialty area since her first day of practice. She submitted a story about a day in her life as nurse. As you can see, she has not only survived but thrived during her first year:

*From a deep sleep I heard a familiar tune going off. I slowly opened my eyes and realized it was my alarm clock. I woke up, got ready, and left home for my journey. It was a sunny morning, a perfect day to be spent at the beach, but that was not where I was headed. As a nurse, I miss many sunny days, many holidays, and many family reunions, but all for a good purpose. As soon as I walked into the hospital, I forgot how nice it was outside. I was now in my own little world and ready to begin another day where I knew I was going to make a difference in someone's life.*

*As usual I arrived in the unit early, got ready for report, and began my shift. I looked at my assignment and realized that I had two new patients I had never taken care of; one was an oncology patient and the other a bone marrow transplant patient, KG. Thoughts began racing through my mind. I had no idea what to expect. I began to look into KG's report sheet, MAR, Caredex, and asked one of her primary physicians to tell me a little bit more about her.*

*From the report sheet I learned that KG had a very busy night. I found out she was going to need packed red blood cells that morning and she normally gets premedicated prior to blood transfusions. My heart began pounding, thinking it was going to be a crazy day. I was embarking on a new mission. After I finished taking the report, I calmly walked to the patient's bedside computer and printed out her lab sheet. I then felt I had sufficient information and knowledge to care for this patient.*

*Later that morning, by 8 a.m., a tall woman with long hair and a dazzling smile approached me at the nurse station desk and introduced herself as KG's mom. I told her I was KG's nurse for the day and asked, "Is there anything I can do to help you?" With concern in her tone she said, "My daughter does not feel well." I walked in the room and there rested a young and beautiful little girl. She looked pale and needed a blow of oxygen to help her breathe more comfortably. I introduced myself and touched her fragile hand, and she gave me a quick, hopeful smile. I went ahead and rechecked KG's blood pressure, and now it was 88/31 with MAP of 50. Her oxygen saturation was 97%, with blow-by oxygen, and she did not look in any distress. I checked her pulses, which were strong and regular, her skin was warm to the touch. I did a neurologic check, and it was also within normal limits. I told her mom that I would continue to monitor KG's blood pressure and her assessment was stable. Furthermore, I told her I would notify the team about KG's low blood pressure. As promised, I went to notify a physician about KG's condition and none of them were available; they had gone to see a patient who was in the ICU. I went back into the room to see KG and rechecked her blood pressure; it was still low, 90's/20's. Even though the patient did not look in any distress, her low blood pressure alarmed me. It was the first time I had a patient with such low blood pressure. I learned about hypotension in nursing school but never had a patient who experienced it. In my mind I said, "Oh my God, I hope she does not code." I calmed myself down and confirmed that the patient was not having any difficulty breathing. I surveyed the room to make sure that all the emergency equipment was in the room and the call light was within the mom's reach. I encouraged her mom to call me as I stepped out of the room to go talk to the charge nurse because I did not feel comfortable with my patient's blood pressure so low.*

After a year on a specialty unit, Neusas is consistently assessing the status of patients and recognizes her intuitive feelings of discomfort. She knows to request a colleague to be another set of eyes and ears to confirm her concerns. Neusa built on her past experience on the unit. She recognizes the necessity of notifying the physician and feels comfortable calling the doctor. She again listened to her intuition and anticipates the possibility of a code. So many things to consider:

*I explained the situation to the charge nurse and asked her to go in with me to reassess the patient. As the charge nurse was assessing the patient, I rechecked the blood pressure and it remained low, 80's/30's. Both the charge nurse and I agreed that the patient's blood pressure was low, but she was perfusing well and we would continue to monitor the patient's blood pressure closely. Mom was not satisfied with that answer. I remained with the patient and mother and the charge nurse went to page the doctors. A few minutes later the whole team walked in the room and began to assess the patient, and I rechecked her blood pressure. Her blood pressure was low in the supine position. KG said she needed to go to the bathroom. As I assisted her to the bathroom, the team engaged in a conversation with the mom explaining that the patient was stable and they were going to transfuse her for her low hematocrit and that would help bring her blood pressure up. After the transfusion, the plan was for the patient to receive Lasix, which would in turn help her respiratory status.*

*As KG got back into bed I rechecked her blood pressure and now it was 105/56 with a MAP of 69; oxygen saturation was 94% on room air. Mom smiled and looked relieved. I encouraged the patient to sit up, which was going to help her breath better on her own, and it could also help to stabilize her blood pressure when she was awake and alert.*

*As I was busy with the patient, the RN-in-charge and the training RN-in-charge ordered the blood, primed the tubing, and got the premedication ready so I could infuse the medications as soon as possible.*

*As I reflected back on the shift, I recognized that I felt supported in every way and did not feel alone. In case an emergency was to occur, I knew I could count on my colleagues to help me provide the best type of care for my patient. My quiet and normal day did not feel the same any longer. Even though it was only 10 a.m. it felt like 4 p.m. A lot was done in this short period of time. Although the family dynamics were difficult, given the fact that the parents, particularly the mom, asked many questions and had certain expectations, I felt I had delivered good quality care and used my delegation skills well. I felt, in my first year of practice, I had grown intellectually and professionally and because of this I was now able to maintain myself calmly in order to think critically through the situation, assess the patient appropriately, and delegate skills as needed. In this moment, I was no longer a naive new graduate but a competent nurse who was using her resources and providing the best type of care to her patient and family. With the charge nurses' help, the team orders, my assessment, and nursing interventions, by the evening KG was feeling better and had gotten out of bed to do syringe painting in the hall. It is amazing how a quiet and calm day can change in seconds and how numerous events can happen simultaneously.*

Neusa recognizes her progress as an experienced nurse, using her delegation skills, feeling supported by her colleagues, keeping her cool, and managing care on the individual and family level. She has come a long way in just a year.

Kim had another kind of experience altogether. She was frustrated by the lack of teamwork, the minimal support, and the absence of an esprit de corps. Kim is a bright, assertive nurse who has worked in a CCU for a year. This is her take on the scene:

*The sheer responsibility of being an RN is shocking, although there is no prestige with the responsibility. It's just shocking how much nurses actually do. It takes so much from you emotionally, physically, and mentally.*

*In addition, there is definitely horizontal violence of back stabbing, competition in report, and showing you up in front of the new preceptees. It takes so much energy to be constantly on your guard. We are still referred to as "these new grads," which I always find demeaning.*

*It is not the norm here to feel like you have given good patient care. The norm is: no break, no food, no pee. This place feels like it is a badge of honor not to take a break. In fact, I feel guilty if I do take a break and I get looks from people.*

*Every time I go in I have to prove myself. The MDs do not have to prove themselves; they are the doctors and that is accepted. This is like a dysfunctional family. There is a rigid hierarchy. The attending says to the residents and nurses, "You guys run the unit." It is just pretending that we are all on a team. Older nurses just bark orders: "You need to do this!"*

*Still I recognize that as you build confidence, you compare and contrast with sound reasoning behind it. There is a science, but it is very gray. There is no one right way; there are a dozen different ways to do it. Now I ask for feedback. I have to be proactive.*

Patient care can definitely be challenging, but with collaborative teamwork, educational resources, and preceptor support, a work environment that empowers nurses can be created. The majority of nurses who we interviewed felt they worked in supportive environments. Some witnessed bullying behavior and learned to work around unsupportive colleagues. Others, like Kim, recognized the culture of the whole unit as dysfunctional. All of the reports of intimidating behavior came from nurses who had been bright, competent students with an optimistic view of their future career. The work environment changed their attitude.

Although this problem of bullying has been recognized and progress has been made in educating nurses about the deleterious effects of such negative behavior, nurses still report that some select staff continue to intimidate newer nurses. You and I know that our caring profession cannot tolerate such uncaring behavior. Horizontal violence undermines the nurse's confidence and is demoralizing. Nursing turnover, lowered confidence, and a decrease in morale ultimately will affect patient safety. There needs to be zero-tolerance policies on each unit. Every unit must have a procedure for managing this unprofessional behavior. *Do not* tolerate intimidation. Speak up, find an ally, go to your preceptor, inform the nurse manager. If you feel there is not an adequate response, look for another position. Individual burnout is most often the result of system problems. If the system problem of intimidation is not confronted, do not stick around for burnout to become part of your attitude. You are too valuable.

Liz, after a year in practice on a specialty unit in a different facility, has a very different story:

*Everyone helps you out here, the residents, the attending, dietary, the lab, and the CNAs. It is all about teamwork. We are in this together. We have board rounds, where we all meet together to figure out the next step with the patient. As a team we talk about ethical issues, and each of us feels comfortable expressing our different opinions.*

*I wanted to work in an inner city with diverse groups of patients. It is exciting and challenging. This morning I had an adolescent mom from Somalia, this afternoon a young Hispanic mom. Many of our patients come from shelters because of domestic violence. They look up to the nurses. I do so much teaching from how to hold a baby to how to breastfeed. I love my job! But I am thinking about grad school . . . I want to learn more.*

Throughout our interview Liz kept emphasizing the importance of critical thinking: "You can learn anything but you need to be critically thinking all the time, questioning, communicating, advocating for your patients and yourself. I speak up for myself all the time. If the assignment is overwhelming I tell them, so we can redistribute or get some help."

Tammi also went right into a specialty. She accepted a position on the same unit where she had done her senior internship, where she knew there was a team of nurses she enjoyed working with. She chose to stay in a small community hospital where the nurses do everything so she could learn complete patient care.

*It has been almost a year since I started my job as an RN in the childbirth center. A lot has changed since then I'm sure, but I can't help but wonder how far I have actually progressed. Just when I think I am in a comfortable place of skill and knowledge, I get knocked back by something new that I've never seen and have no idea how to handle. Luckily I have a great team around me, and whenever I get stuck they are readily available to help. Because my hospital is a small community hospital, the nurses in the childbirth center do everything. We do labor and delivery, postpartum care, and nursery care for sick babies. I have been able to work in the OR for C-sections, put an IV in a newborn, take care of GYN patients who have just had hysterectomies, and teach breastfeeding. That is just a small sample of the diverse jobs I have on this unit.*

*I have never given birth, but I have learned to see that as an advantage. I can't say, "Well, when I had my baby, I did this or I thought that." I have no prejudgments about they best way to do things. But I have seen hundreds of women go through this amazing experience in their own way, and I support them in the way they want to be supported, not how I think they should be supported. I wouldn't even know what that is.*

*Recently I realized that I have been operating from a task-only perception. I go into a room with a checklist in my head trying not to forget everything I have to do. I am now starting to see the big picture of tasks, personal relationships, and comforting the patient. I am remembering that I can use the skills I have learned to help me in this job. I can use acupressure and meditation to help my patients and form the kind of practice I would like to have. This was a really big step for me, but I know with time I'll be practicing the way I wanted to when I first came to nursing school.*

*After a year I still feel like a new nurse. Insecurities have not departed. I recently had a nightmare that I was in the operating room setting up for a C-section and I couldn't open a package correctly. I had to keep doing it over and over again with everyone yelling at me that I was incompetent. I still have those feelings in the back of my subconscious, and they creep in now and again. I am giving those feelings of inadequacy some space to vent and then reminding myself that I have accomplished so much in this last year. But it is hard to see my triumphs when the failures overshadow them. Hopefully those feelings will subside. Advice from other nurses in this field reassure me that I am not alone with these thoughts, and it takes a good 5 years in this specialty to become an expert nurse. So I'll let you know how that goes.*

A year out, confidence, insecurities, good communication, and lack of voice are all predictable parts of the first-year experience. As you can hear from the stories on the front line, the responses of the new nurse run the gamut of feeling confident one day to overwhelmed the next. Fortunately, hospitals and educational programs are recognizing the importance of supporting the new nurse with programs designed to pick up where school left off. Hospitals recognize that preceptors should not just be recruited to mentor new nurses and then leave them on their own. There are now programs to train preceptors in the art of coaching new nurses, with recognition, supervisor support, and sometimes financial remuneration.

The expectations during your first year are high, the work is critical, and you will have an incredibly important role in a health-care system—a system that needs a lot of repair. You will be on the inside, in a position to know what works and what does not. You are entering nursing just at the right time when nursing work is valued and publicly recognized as essential. The nurse is at the hub of the wheel of the health-care team. Don't let anyone tell you differently. Never underestimate your influence.

If you feel your influence flagging, your voice suppressed, or your work going unrecognized, speak up and let your supervisor know. If you do not feel heard, consider moving to a place that will value your work, appreciate your input, and recognize nursing's critical contribution to patient care. All nurses should be recognized and rewarded for their work. You can start by recognizing other nurses. Let your preceptor know what you appreciate, give a peer positive feedback, and be a team player yourself. So many nurses who made suggestions for the first year out said, "Be a team player." I know you feel brand new with little to offer, but when you've finished your assignment you can ask your colleagues if they'd like assistance. You can locate evidence from the literature readily and you can express your opinion too.

One participant in the *First Year Study* described the best thing about nursing:

*It has all these different aspects that speak to a whole bunch of parts of you. You have to be able to communicate, there's a definite art to it. There's also a science to it, it's very task oriented. You have to be very organized, but you have to be kind and considerate, a people person. You have to be everything. I like that. I like being everything. I go home at the end of the day, continually amazed at how many times a week patients and families tell me, "You're a really great nurse." It is a nice feeling to be completely appreciated for the work that you do.*

The other side is that the worst part about nursing is when you have to be everything and you're just not in the mood:

*Even when I don't want to talk to my patient anymore, I still have to. I want to say, "I wish I could give you better care, but you're really annoying." It is not easy to care for someone with a difficult personality. It's so hard to give good care because you don't want to go into the room. Makes me feel really guilty. And it's exhausting.*

Look for resources in your facility. Amanda, who worked nights in a small community hospital, had a clinical resource nurse on every shift. Jane had a clinical nurse specialist assigned to her unit. Megan joined her professional organization, American Psychiatric Nurses Association, for the student rate of $25, right before she graduated. Professional organizations have so much to offer. You can get as involved as you like, serve on a committee, run for office, or attend a local or national conference. I can guarantee you will be inspired by your nurse colleagues, learn about new evidence, and network with peers and potential mentors. Besides, it's fun to travel, get away from work, and visit a place you have not been before. What's not to like?

# CONCLUSION

You will find a work environment that supports you and you will be an assertive advocate for your patients. That means you will build your practice on evidence, be actively involved in representing your profession at the local and national level through hospital committee work, attending conferences, and being involved in your professional organization. You will make nursing proud, move health care forward, and have your patients say how pleased they are to have you as their nurse. You will make it through your first year and you will celebrate when you get there! How's that for positive affirmations? Thinking positively, being smart about yourself and your organization, and learning every day are what is going to get you from here to there. As Dr. Clifford said, "You are like a precious jewel, and don't let anyone tell you otherwise!"

# [CHAPTER 10]

# Where to Next?

*"Once social change begins, it cannot be reversed. You cannot uneducate the person who has learned to read. You cannot humiliate the person who feels pride. You cannot oppress the people who are not afraid anymore. We have seen the future, and the future is ours."*

—Cesar Chavez

What is your future now that you are an accomplished nurse? Is it time for a new population of patients or a different unit, another shift, or a promotion? Are you ready for a different location? Or, are you thinking about grad school? There are so many possibilities. In this chapter let's consider your options. This chapter is a little different from the rest in that it is packed with factual information designed to assist you in sorting out your future choices. The facts may seem a bit tedious, but they paint a broad picture of what your options are. If you are considering moving within your current hospital system or specialty certification or heading off to grad school, you will need all the facts. You want to make the right move for the right reason, don't you agree?

A career move should be well planned so the time and energy to make such a step fits your interests. So what color is your parachute? Do you know that book? Richard N. Bolles first published *What Color Is Your Parachute?*" in 1970. Bolles (2009) explains that he came up with the title in response to friends who would tell him they wanted to bail out of their job. His response was "What color is your parachute?" Sounds to me like he was encouraging them to look around and develop a plan for landing. Now, because it is predicted that everyone will have at least three changes of a career in their lifetime, a new, updated version of the parachute book's practical advice on job hunting comes out every year.

You already know you are passionate about patient care and skilled in providing nursing care, so we don't have to start at the beginning, but we could look around and see what is out there. Where do you want to land? A step up the clinical ladder? A radical geographic move? A BS to PhD program? These are great choices. Let's start with staying in the place you now work and surveying promotion possibilities, improving your skills, and broadening your knowledge base through certification.

# CLINICAL LADDERS

Clinical ladders are career advancement programs designed to recognize and reward excellence in nursing through progression and promotion. Many facilities offer a version of a clinical ladder program to encourage skilled nurses to stay at the bedside while being recognized and rewarded for the good work that they do. Historically, to be promoted in hospitals, a nurse would have to move into a staff education or a nurse manager position. These limited choices encourage the nurse with patient care experience to move away from the bedside in order to increase earning power. With the advent of clinical ladders, competent nurses are rewarded for direct patient care.

Clinical ladder programs generally have levels, clinical nurse 1,2,3, etc., where each step has an increased level of responsibility that may include specialty certification, professional organization involvement, or formal education. The advancement programs are designed to recognize nurses who have excelled in clinical practice, leadership, and professionalism. For example, the Staff Nurse III/IV in Kaiser Permanente's clinical ladder level is described as follows:

The Staff Nurse III/IV and HH/H III functions in the clinical setting as an exemplary caregiver to patients, a model of proficiency for coworkers, and a colleague to physicians. From years of nursing experience and a continued expansion of clinical knowledge, the Clinical Expert (SN III/IV or HH/H III) is a skilled practitioner who demonstrates leadership by:

1. Identifying, communicating, and fulfilling patient needs
2. Coordinating and utilizing facility and community resources to meet patient needs
3. Promoting a multidisciplinary approach to patient care

4. Assuming a teaching-coaching role with other nurses and health-team members, and

5. Maintaining a flexible approach to resource constraints (http://nursingpathways .kp.org/ncal/careers/ladders/index.html)

There is no standard clinical ladder program. Each facility designs a career advancement opportunity that fits with its organizational mission and patient care needs. One program emphasizes knowledge, judgment, experience, and leadership while another focuses on education, research, and evidence-based practice. Some programs encourage nursing involvement on hospital committees, in local nursing organizations, and at the national conference level. Applicants to clinical ladder programs typically submit a portfolio that includes annual evaluations, peer reviews, and a clinical narrative description of a practice situation. Portfolio preparation classes may be available at your facility. In addition, there are several hospital Web sites that describe and give examples of clinical narratives. Just Google "clinical nurse narratives" to read motivating exemplars. Take advantage of such promotional support through in-house classes and online information. It can be helpful to compare and contrast your work with nurses on other units. Once the portfolio application is complete, a committee of peers and expert nurses may interview the candidates to develop recommendations for promotion.

Overall, clinical ladder programs are rated positively by staff and administration. They have been shown to have an effect on retention and job satisfaction, which ultimately produces cost savings through deceased turnover. Programs that facilitate nursing leadership and promote professional development result in a win-win situation for the organization and the individual nurse. Organizations are proud to have expert nurses at the bedside, recognizing that they contribute to quality improvement, patient safety, and patient satisfaction. So, if you have not looked into promotional possibilities yet, find out the criteria for your facility's clinical ladder program. It is important to be recognized for your work. Some clinical ladder levels require specialty certification.

# CERTIFICATION

Certification, as defined by the American Board of Nursing Specialties (ABNS) (2005), is "the formal recognition of the specialized knowledge, skills, and experience demonstrated by the achievement of standards identified by a nursing specialty to promote optimal health outcomes" (http://www.nursingcertification.org/). Through an exam, certification recognizes increased knowledge and expertise from the basic nursing license. Although state licensure provides assurance that the nurse meets the minimal requirements for safe practice and the legal authority for an individual to practice professional nursing, certification indicates increased competency. Certification recognizes an individual nurse has successfully passed a certification exam to earn the credential that demonstrates specialized knowledge, skills, and experience. After meeting defined eligibility criteria and successful completion of the exam, the certification candidate achieves a nationally recognized credential.

Certification is not required for practice but may be a stipulation for promotion. The American Nurses Credentialing Center (ANCC) suggests that board certification and recognition empowers nurses to contribute to better patient care. ANCC, a subsidiary of the American Nurses Association, is one of the organizations that offers certification exams and credentialing. The ANCC's certification and portfolio recognition programs validate nurses' skills, knowledge, and abilities. Recognition of nurse expertise is believed to produce better practitioners. The results of several studies conducted by credentialing organizations have indicated that certification provides a positive benefit to patient care quality, patient safety, and nursing performance.

Certification of expertise aids the profession and protects the public. Encouragement and recognition of expertise by practicing, studying, and passing the exam benefits the individual nurse. Having the certification credential on your name badge enables the public to identify nursing competence. Thus, certification is a formal process that recognizes specialization, enhances professionalism, and can serve as a criterion for financial reimbursement. ANCC reports that board-certified nurses are in the greatest demand and do command the highest salaries. It has been reported that certified nurses earn an average of $9,000 more than their counterparts who are not board certified. ANCC reports that certification is accepted by governing boards, insurers, and the military. Consult the ANCC Web site for a listing of certification exams, www.nursecredentialing.org/. To sit for a certification examination, you must have:

- A current registered nurse license
- Documentation that you have the appropriate educational requirements
- Relevant experience in the specialty field

Once you have met the eligibility requirements, you can then register to take the certification examination.

One last piece of information: Certificate programs are different than certification. A certificate may be awarded at the end of a continuing education program or for an in-house education offer indicating program completion, but a certificate does not necessarily mean specialty or expertise certification. A certificate *is not* a certification. To move into an advanced role to function as an advanced practice registered nurse (APRN), both graduate education and certification credentialing are required.

# ADVANCED PRACTICE REGISTERED NURSE

Specific graduate school programs can provide you with the education to sit for a certification exam to become an advanced practice registered nurse (APRN). An APRN is educated in one of the four roles: certified registered nurse anesthetist (CRNA), certified nurse midwife (CNM), clinical nurse specialist (CNS), and certified nurse practitioner (CNP). Within an accredited educational program, APRNs focus on at least one of the six populations: family/individual across the lifespan, adult gerontology, pediatrics, neonatal, women's health/gender-related, or psych/mental health. The common coursework in every APRN graduate program are advanced physiology/pathophysiology, advanced health assessment, and advanced pharmacology. These core courses run concurrently with graduate-level clinical experiences. Each program incorporates specialty knowledge and a role development course, a theoretical basis for advanced nursing, and a research component emphasizing translational research. Translational research may encompass being part of a research team, evaluating evidence, and translating research into practice. At the end of the program, graduates sit for a certification exam that assesses national competencies of the APRN core, competencies of the role, and at least one population focus area. The advanced practice registered nurse is prepared to assume responsibility for health promotion and health maintenance, assessment, diagnosis, and management of health problems including prescriptive privileges for pharmacologic and nonpharmacologic interventions. The functions of the four APRN roles are as follows:

1. The certified registered nurse anesthetist (CRNA) is prepared to provide anesthesia care across the lifespan. The patient's health

ranges from healthy to severely ill. Anesthesia care can be provided in diverse settings, including hospitals, dental offices, podiatry, ophthalmology, plastic surgeons' suites, or in U.S. military public health hospitals. CRNAs are the primary anesthesia providers in rural America, enabling health-care facilities in these medically underserved areas to offer obstetrical, surgical, and trauma stabilization services. In some states, CRNAs are the sole providers in nearly 100% of the rural hospitals.

When anesthesia is administered by a nurse anesthetist, it is recognized as the practice of nursing; when administered by an anesthesiologist, it is recognized as the practice of medicine. Regardless of whether their educational background is in nursing or medicine, all anesthesia professionals give anesthesia the same way.

2. The certified nurse midwife (CNM) provides primary health care for women across the lifespan, including preconception, prenatal, childbirth, postpartum care, and care of the newborn. The CNM can provide family planning, gynecologic care, and care for the woman's partner as they are related to reproductive health and sexually transmitted diseases. Midwifery care is provided in diverse settings such as in the home, the hospital, a birth center, or an ambulatory care setting.

3. The clinical nurse specialist (CNS) integrates care across the continuum through the patient, nurse, or organization. The goal of the CNS is to improve patient outcomes and nursing care by consulting on individual patient care, mentoring the individual nurse, and empowering the nursing group to make system changes that will facilitate ethical decision making to alleviate patient distress and promote health. The CNS works in a variety of settings that include unit-based and systems-based roles.

4. The certified nurse practitioner (CNP) provides care across the wellness-illness continuum through direct primary and acute care across settings. CNPs are prepared to diagnose and treat individuals with undifferentiated symptoms providing assessment and ongoing and comprehensive care. NP care includes health promotion, disease prevention, health education, and counseling in hospitals, clinics, offices, schools, and in their own private practice.

How do you decide when to make the leap from work back to school? After 3 years of practice on a specialty unit, Neusa decided to return to grad school for an advanced practice degree. She writes,

*Becoming a nurse was an ideal that I decided to pursue during my sophomore year. In 2006, I was able to fulfill that goal and enter the nursing profession. I have been practicing for almost 3 years in the Bone Marrow Transplant Unit. The best thing about being a nurse is that despite how sick the patient may be, as a nurse I will always find a way to touch his or her life and advocate for both patient and family. In order to provide patients and families with the best quality of care, I felt I wanted to learn more; that is why obtaining a graduate degree is of great importance to me.*

*Throughout my life, my family has always encouraged me to pursue a higher education. Even before I completed my bachelor's degree, I knew that I wanted to continue to pursue a graduate degree in nursing. The advancement of technology, the complexity of clinical care, and the demand for highly-skilled individuals in the workplace require more than a bachelor's degree. After being a nurse for almost 2 years, I began to question things. It was not like when I was a new graduate and was focused so much on the nursing task. At this stage, I wanted to know more about the disease process, new medications, research, and wanted to know how I could best take care of my patients. After all the questioning, I had an answer. "I am young, I don't have any kids, my husband is also in school. It is time to go back to school." I decided to go back to school to get my MSN and become a pediatric nurse practitioner. Once I earn a master's degree I will be able to improve myself and help others in my community. My hope upon completing the master's program is to provide primary care to a diverse population, and help eliminate health disparities in my community. I will also have the opportunity to further involve myself in improving the health-care system and educating future generations of nurses. Learning never stops. Why wait to advance your degree later when you can do it now? The power is in our hands. We just have to keep being motivated.*

Virginia Henderson cited the same reasons as Neusa when she was asked why a nurse should go back to school. "The desire to learn more, to improve your ability to contribute to patient care" was Miss Henderson's answer. Miss Henderson is described as the most famous nurse of the twentieth century. Read her inspiring biographical statement on Sigma Theta Tau's library Web site, www.nursinglibrary.org. I had the good fortune to meet Miss Henderson when, at 92 years of age, she came to speak at our university. I drove down to New Haven to pick up Miss Henderson at her well-appointed apartment, furnished with beautiful antiques and a concert piano. We had plenty of time to chat during the 2-hour car ride.

Back on campus we were greeted by a standing-room-only auditorium packed with over 200 alums, students, and faculty. Following her awe-inspiring lecture, a student asked how much schooling a nurse should have. Miss Henderson was quick to respond with a timeless answer: "A nurse should have as much education as possible so she or he is better equipped to meet the needs of a broad variety and diversity of patients." End of story.

So it is not surprising to hear the same theme in the narratives in this chapter: more nurse education, more comprehensive patient care. Bridget worked as an RN in a clinic practice where she could see the necessity for advanced knowledge, increased responsibility, and a higher level of practice for herself

*When I was working as an RN, in a school health center, I was learning from the physician and the nurse practitioner. I saw dozens of students and triaged what needed to be seen by the MD or NP. I used standing orders to treat problems as fully as I could before sending patients to appointments. In doing so, I found that I was mimicking the NP as closely as possible by doing in-depth exams that were beyond my training as an RN. I loved using the standing orders to diagnose a UTI or strep throat and get the students the antibiotics they needed by using my own judgment. It became clear to me that I wanted the ability to make the decisions myself, to have greater responsibility, and to have the knowledge that a higher level of practice required. I admired the nurse practitioners whom I worked with, and I imagined that I could do what they were doing. They encouraged me to pursue my goal.*

Currently, APRNs can be educated at the masters or doctoral level. In addition to the APRN option, there are programs that offer a master's in nursing education, nursing administration/management, and a clinical nurse leader (CNL) degree. A master's in education will prepare you to be a clinical instructor with a core curriculum in theory and research with focused educational courses and elective options to fit your individual interests. A degree in management is similar, with core courses in theory and research, management courses, and the opportunity to take electives in other disciplines such as women's studies, sociology, public health, or management.

The CNL is a degree that enlarges the nurse-at-the-bedside scope of practice. The CNL is not an advanced practice role or administrative role. The focus of the curriculum is on nursing leadership, clinical outcomes management, and care environment management. CNL programs have been developed in partnership with the practice environment so the graduate is prepared at a level designed by the collaboration of practice and education. As a CNL you would be able to direct patient care at the unit level in a variety of health-care settings through the integration of patient care evaluation, team performance facilitation, and evidence-based practice. The practice focus is on improving patient safety, increasing quality health outcomes, and facilitating organizational system functioning. The CNL is a vital role in the development of creative solutions for our future health-care system. Different CNL programs offer different emphases on specific health-care concerns. For example, one program's focus is on health promotion, risk reduction, disease prevention, and illness management; another focus may be on evaluating client outcomes, assessing cohort risk, and functioning as part of an interdisciplinary team. All CNL students are expected to function across clinical settings to meet the demands of a complex care delivery system while supervising the application of research evidence and the efficient use of resources to effect organizational change. The CNL is a provider and a manager at the point of care for a specific group of individuals and cohorts, assuming accountability for the outcomes of the clients. The CNL graduate is expected to lead, coordinate, delegate, and evaluate care provided by the health-care team. The white paper on the American Association of Colleges of Nursing (AACN) Web site gives a very thorough picture of the background, expectations, and future of the CNL role (www.aacn.nche.edu/CNL/)

Cara decided to go back to school for a CNL degree to complement a rewarding and diverse career. She writes,

*Nurses assume essential roles of practice that include providing, teaching, managing, and leading. Nurses function within legal/ethical boundaries and provide an environment that supports individuality, cultural diversity, mutual respect, and dignity. Each graduate course I completed helped me to rediscover the role of a nurse and brought me back to the core values that I treasured so much in my earlier nursing years. This reinforced my decision to continue my education. It coincided with my desire to have a positive impact at some level.*

*After I graduated with my CNL I was employed as a clinical nurse educator at a large teaching facility. My role is a joint venture with a Research 1 university where I am a clinical faculty coordinator for a health assessment course. I work with experienced nurses, new nurses, and student nurses. I oversee a pilot clinical model for nursing students, the designated educational unit (DEU), which has just successfully completed its second clinical semester.*

*I facilitate interdisciplinary workshops with medical students and nursing students as a way to improve communication among the members of the healthcare team. I serve as a member to various hospital committees to help ensure quality performance, maintain certifications, and continuing education units specific to my role and teach a cardiac dysrhythmia course for multiple hospitals. I have been invited to speak at neighboring hospitals regarding nurses as mentors to their leadership team. I feel like I'm living the dream! At a recent meeting with the chief nurse officer of the hospital, I stated that I am fortunate to do what I love and get a paycheck!*

*Recently, a physician, who is familiar with the financial rewards that my former work in a medical device company afforded, commented on the fact that I left such a lucrative position. He was surprised I would "give up" so much. I responded that I have come to learn how much I have gained in my new endeavor. I followed my instinct and truly feel that I belong right where I am. I can't imagine any greater feeling toward my career. I am wealthy, in fact, far wealthier than many in gratification, not to mention a plethora of new knowledge to explore and to motivate me. And most astounding to me is the sense of paying something forward.*

How is that for enthusiasm? Although Cara had a diverse career to begin with, the CNL degree opened up many new possibilities.

In 2004, the member schools of the AACN voted to endorse the move of education for advanced nursing practice from the master's degree to a doctor of nursing practice (DNP) by 2015. AACN wrote a white paper covering the history and future necessity for a doctoral level of practice. On their Web site they also offer the essentials for a DNP program. Both will help you determine if this is the right path for you (visit www.aacn.nche.edu). Beth, already practicing as a CNP, decided on a doctorate in nursing practice. She is pursuing a DNP in the psych/mental health track:

*When I graduated with my BS in nursing I did so almost by default. I didn't really know if I wanted to be a nurse but figured I would have a job while I decided what I wanted to do. If someone would have told me at that time that I would go back to school in nursing, not once but twice, I would never have believed them. But after trying several areas in nursing, I fell in love with psychiatric nursing.*

*Working as a hospital psych nurse, however, only carried me so far. After having been in that role for several years, I felt that I had reached the level that I could. I knew I didn't want to be in management, but I wanted something more. I started hearing about nurse practitioners. At first I thought I would go into a family NP program because it would be more practical. But I kept being drawn back to my real passion for psych and decided to go with what I was excited about instead of what seemed practical.*

*My timing was not good, and life events slowed my progress, but 11 days after my youngest child was born, I defended my thesis, completing my program, and I graduated with my MS, entering the work force as a psychiatric mental health nurse practitioner. As I said, I love being in practice, so at that time I figured I had reached the end of my needs for education.*

*I was wrong. I have loved being a psych NP more than I hoped I would. I truly believe I am one of the lucky people who has managed to find themselves in a career they truly love. But once again life changed the plan on me. Soon after I graduated my MS program and started working as an NP, the buzz word in NP preparation changed to DNP. I didn't think much of it personally at first, but after 5 years in practice, feeling more comfortable in my role as an NP, I became restless—not for a change in practice, but for a change in level of practice. And so I am now entering my final year in a DNP program. I am not changing specialty or profession, but feel this will enable me to bring my practice to a higher level. I want to not only offer my patients the highest level of care, but also to be stimulated in my own intellectual pursuits in practice. An exciting aspect of graduate school is more than just what you learn directly. It is a lot about how you think and how you learn and explore knowledge. I already find myself thinking of what I could do with more education in the future, but don't tell my children!*

The doctorate of nursing practice builds on the master's requirements with the addition of an emphasis on in-depth study of quality improvement, informatics, leadership, and research translation. The DNP is practice focused as opposed to the PhD where conducting research is the primary emphasis. For both degrees there are different entry points. Both the DNP and PhD have a post-master's entry and now many programs offer a BS-DNP or BS-PhD. The AACN's Web site, www.aacn.nche.edu, has descriptions of the history, rationale, and requirements for both types of doctoral programs.

It is important to consider how the expectations of each degree fit with your future career. Many nurses shy away from the research aspect of the PhD degree and choose a more familiar practice option that fits with their career goals. Think carefully about which route will lead you to the end you have in mind. Are you thinking of being a tenured university faculty member, teaching classes and conducting research? Or are you considering functioning in a primary care position, being an expert clinician and translating research into practice on the front line?

Sheila, a recent BS graduate and a year into the PhD program, writes,

*When I was a little girl I knew that someday I would grow up to be a doctor. Little did I know that this doctorate would be in nursing. I had no idea this degree even existed. I never knew a nurse, and as I struggled through my undergraduate years to form myself into one; I felt I was missing something. I had been called to nursing in my sophomore year. At that time I believed that I chose it because it would be easy and pay well. Wow, was I wrong. I was an honors student throughout my undergraduate years, and while I was in the minority in my graduating class, I added extra classes and a research project to my busy senior year. After this experience I felt like I had found the thing I was missing. I would not be "just a nurse." I would solve the problems of the world of nursing. Well, this is probably overambitious, but you get the idea. I could not rejoin the majority and jump out into the world of practice unarmed to answer these daunting questions. And so, here I am, finishing my first full year of PhD study. Already I find myself looking differently at the practice world around me. For example, I have learned to see what would appear to be annoying nit-picking behavior from some of my elderly patients as a self-management strategy. I have learned to speak with my supervisors and supervisees as colleagues and collaborate with them to solve the small problems of my residents. All of this in my first year and a half of nursing practice! It sounds much more ambitious on paper than it feels to me. To me it just feels right. As much as I love being "just a nurse," I know that in being more I can do more for my patients and for the world of nursing.*

Can you hear the echo of Virginia Henderson's words? "A nurse should have as much education as possible so she or he is better equipped to meet the needs of a broad variety and diversity of patients." When narratives started coming in that related to why nurses decided to go back to graduate school, four common themes stood out:

- Feeling like there must be more to nursing
- Experiencing the need to advance their own practice
- Developing research knowledge

- Discovering a path that offered a broader and more in-depth view of nursing that would lead to a higher level of patient care

Lisa went directly from a second bachelor's program to a BS to PhD track:

*My journey to graduate nursing happened unexpectedly. As I was finishing a second bachelor's program, I was interested but did not have a plan to pursue a graduate degree just yet. When my faculty advisor asked me at the completion of the capstone project I had worked on as part of the undergraduate honor program, "Why aren't you applying to graduate school?" it provided the jump-start I needed.*

*I love being in the PhD program because it has exposed me to the world of nursing knowledge and that knowledge informs my practice as a community nurse in significant ways (significant to my experience as a human and a nurse and I hope significant to my clients). I feel very privileged to be able to live the experience with my graduate student colleagues, and to continue learning from my course work, faculty adviser, and the other nursing faculty.*

*As to why now? In my personal life, I can only reply, "why not now"? I worked for a number of years in local and regional government and that work was challenging but not fulfilling. Graduate school has afforded me the opportunity to work in a variety of settings and focus energy on developing knowledge. Every day I am engaged in learning. Working with people, particularly older adults, has always been my passion, and now it is my specialty. Graduate work provides an opportunity to contribute positively to the health of older adults. What a great way to spend time and effort!*

Carolyn traveled a route from a BS to PhD that included managing the life/work balance:

*What made me consider returning to school and why now? Great questions . . . and ones I ask myself multiple times during the semester, typically "what was I thinking going back to school?" Several reasons come to mind, each as important as the other. I've always loved to learn, and there is so much to learn about. A terminal degree would open more doors; I would have more choices. I've taught adults and have loved it. A PhD would qualify me to teach in a college/university. I'm a nerd; I love the classroom. September equals back to school and new notebooks and texts and pens . . . and all that cool stuff. This degree would get me into the classroom. And I thought I would have the opportunity to conduct my own research. At the end of the day, however, I think it was just time.*

*I went to college as a married mother. One of my goals upon graduation was to immediately enroll in grad school. I wasn't sure what I wanted from the additional education—just that I wanted it. And life got in the way. My energy went into being a wife and mother and learning how to be an RN. Grad school seemed far away, and honestly, at that point in time, grad school didn't seem pertinent to my life. Time slipped by. Several years after graduation, my life underwent enormous changes. I wasn't ready to consider grad school until several years ago. When my life had finally fallen into a nice rhythm, it seemed to be time to take the idea of grad school from the back burner and examine it. It took me a long time to decide definitively to go back to school. Lots of things to consider. Ugh. Did I want to go through school again? Did I want and could I handle the fatigue now that I was older? What would grad school mean to my relationships? Finances? Could I do this? Was I smart enough to take the GREs to get into a grad school and do the work?*

*I went to an open house at the university one evening—semi spur of the moment. The director of the program was my undergrad psych professor. I found the professor I would be working with was a CNS I had worked with previously. So I felt somewhat comfortable there; I respected these women, and they thought I could do this, so maybe I could. That insecurity (I can't do this . . . am not smart enough and sooner or later one of these smart people is going to figure out that I don't belong here and kick me out) rears its ugly head occasionally. If you do go back, beware 6 weeks into the first semester of study. Don't listen to the voice inside your head telling you your admission was a mistake, you don't belong here, and someone will figure it out and you'll be kicked to the curb. Don't listen. Reach out to your cohorts, they're most likely thinking the same thing, and support each other. Yes, you do belong here.*

*I don't regret my decision to return to school now, over 10 years since pinning. I may not have 30 years of research to look forward to, but I'm different from the woman who graduated from a state college and my research will reflect that professional maturity. I have also met the most incredible, caring, brilliant people at this university. And I have grown in ways I would never have thought possible.*

These decision-making stories are inspirational! Can you see yourself in one? That is the beauty of nursing, there is something for everyone. There are many possibilities for advancement. Choose the path that fits you, whether it is climbing the clinical ladder, a specialty certification, or graduate school. This is a great time to return to school. The profession and the public recognize the need for APNs. Also, there is a staggering faculty shortage, so if you ever considered teaching, now is the time to make the move.

# CONCLUSION

There is an alphabet of choices: CNP, CRNA, CNL, DNP, PhD. You choose. Just as the nurse narratives describe, find a program that suits your needs, supports your interests, provides inspiring role models, and you'll be excited to learn and look forward to practice. There is no question the profession and public need you. You just have to decide when.

## References

American Board of Nursing Specialties (ABNS). (2005). A position statement on the value of specialty nursing certification. Retrieved June 6, 2009, from http:/www.nursingcertification.org.

Bolles, R. N. (2009). *What color is your parachute?* Berkeley, CA: Ten Speed Press.

# APPENDIX

# NCLEX Preparation Resources

## Question Resources

1. *Springhouse NCLEX® Review 4000 CD-ROM* (2008). Philadelphia: Lippincott, Williams & Wilkins. ISBN 13: 978-0781777902.
2. Silvestri, L. (2007). *Saunders Question and Answer Review for NCLEX-RN* (4th ed.). St. Louis: Saunders Elsevier. ISBN 13: 978-1416048503.
3. Saxton, D., Nugent, P., Pelikan, P., & Green, J. (2005). *Mosby's Review Questions for the NCLEX-RN® Examination* (5th ed.). St. Louis: Elsevier, Inc. ISBN 0323024688.
4. *Springhouse NCLEX-RN New Format Questions*. (2008). Philadelphia: Lippincott Williams and Wilkins. ISBN 1-58255-473-0.

## Pharmacology Resources

1. Hogan, M. (Ed.). (2005). *Pharmacology: Reviews and Rationales.* Upper Saddle River, NJ: Prentice Hall. ISBN 013030462X.
2. Waide, L., Roland, B. (2001). *Pharmacology Made Easy for the NCLEX-RN.* Chicago; IL: Chicago Review Press, Incorporated. ISBN 1556523912.
3. Zerwekh, J., Claborn, J., & Gaglione, T. (2005). *Mosby's Pharmacology Memory NoteCards: Visual, Mnemonic and Memory Aids for Nurses.* St. Louis: Mosby Elsevier.
4. Hogan, M., Frandsen, G., Johnson, J., & Warner, L. (2008). *Pharmacology: Reviews & rationales* (2nd ed.). Upper Saddle River, NJ: Pearson Education, Inc. ISBN 13: 978-0-13-243710-3; ISBN 10: 0-13-243710-4.

## Test-Taking Strategies Resources

1. Irwin, B. & Burckhardt, J. (2008). *Kaplan "NCLEX-RN: Strategies for the Registered Nursing Licensing Exam"* 2008-2009.
2. Silvestri, L. (2009). *Saunders Strategies for Test Success: Passing Nursing School and the NCLEX-RN Exam* (2nd ed.). St. Louis: Saunders Elsevier. ISBN 978-1416062028.

3. Irwin, B., & Burckhardt, J. (2010). *NCLEX-RN Exam 2010-2011.* New York: Kaplan. ISBN 978-1419-553448.
4. Hoefler, P. (2008). *Successful Problem Solving and Test-Taking Strategies for Beginning Nursing Students.* Burtonsville, MD: Meds Publishing.
5. Nugent, PM., & Vitale, BA. (2004). *Test Success: Test-Taking Techniques for Beginning Nursing Students* (4th ed.). Philadelphia: FA Davis. ISBN 0-8036-1162-5.
6. Hogan, M. (2008). *Comprehensive Review for NCLEX-RN.* Upper Saddle River, NJ: Pearson Education, Inc. ISBN 13: 978-0-13-119599-8; ISBN 10: 0-13-119599-9.

## Contact Information for NCLEX-RN Preparation Review Courses On Line and/or In-Person

1. Linda Silvestri, 800-598-6730, www.us.elsevierhealth.com/
2. Barbara Murphy, 978-486-3137
3. Kaplan Review Course, 1-800-533-8850

## NCLEX-RN Practice Computer Adaptive Test Simulation

Saxton, D. F., Pelikan, P. K., & Green, J. S. (2004). Mosby's Computer Adaptive Test (CAT) for NCLEX-RN Examination Online (2nd ed.). St. Louis: Mosby. http://www.us.elsevierhealth.com/product. jsp? ISBN 0-32303-252-4

ATI testing—http://www.atitesting.co.

# Index

Note: Page numbers followed by *t* indicate tables; page numbers followed by *f* indicate figures.